BASIC DIAGNOSTIC RADIOLOGY

BASIC DIAGNOSTIC RADIOLOGY

An introductory textbook for students in the medical sciences

Malcolm D. Jones, M.D.

Professor and Vice-Chairman,
Department of Radiology;
Professor of Radiology,
Division of Ambulatory and Community Medicine,
University of California Medical School,
San Francisco, California

Diagrams and drawings by Mrs. Margaret Jones

With 511 illustrations

Saint Louis

The C. V. Mosby Company

1969

To the memory of

Dr. Robert S. Stone

Professor, teacher, and friend

PREFACE

This is not intended to be a definitive text on diagnostic radiology, but is rather an attempt to put into writing the answers to questions most frequently posed by medical students and residents in the various specialties.

Within the past several years, specialized and general textbooks designed to meet the needs of medical students have filled a void that existed for many years. The intention of this work is to provide an introduction for the more expanded texts available to students. Consequently, a distinct emphasis and subsequent concentration is inherent in this book; this intentional type of presentation is an attempt to stress those areas of diagnostic radiology most commonly encountered as well as those topics producing the greatest amount of confusion.

No creative effort such as this is accomplished without the dedicated support of many individuals. I wish to acknowledge the patient and helpfully critical efforts of Mrs. Anneliese Haas and Miss Virginia Voigt, for without their skilled efforts the manuscript could never have been prepared. The staff in the Photography Division of the Communications Office for Research and Training, under the direction of Mr. George T. Vinsant, rose to the challenge of producing a large number of high quality photographs in a short period of time. The unsung heroines of the film file room, Mrs. Bess Patterson and Mrs. Esterline Lacey, with unfailing patience provided me with the tons of raw material from which the illustrations were gleaned. Special acknowledgement is made to my wife, Margaret, for both support and tolerance as well as for her efforts in providing the illustrative art work so necessary in making a book of this type meaningful.

Malcolm D. Jones, M.D.

CONTENTS

BASIC DIAGNOSTIC RADIOLOGY

INTRODUCTION

Summary of basic concepts

The outlines at the beginning of each chapter are intended to provide a concise summary of the subject matter discussed within the chapter. The order of the textual presentation does not lend itself easily to an outline best suited for such a quick review. No attempt has been made, therefore, to limit the summaries to topics elaborated upon in the text or to maintain rigidly the order of presentation.

I. Definition of diagnostic roentgenology

  Production and interpretation of two-dimensional representation of a three-dimensional structure using electromagnetic rays which penetrate the object being studied.

II. Criteria of diagnostic roentgenology

  A. Roentgenographic parameters

    1. Density
    2. Size
    3. Contour
    4. Location
    5. Number
    6. Margination

  B. Roentgenographic appearance of function or form of structure

    1. Valid only at time of recording
    2. May be altered in disease processes

III. Basis of diagnostic roentgenology

  A. Differential absorption of x-rays by various adjoining substances, depending on composition and thickness

  B. That part of x-ray beam passing completely through body recorded on fluoroscope or film

  C. Television image, cineroentgenography, and videotape—all recorded from fluoroscopic screen

  D. Image on x-ray film usually from light from fluorescent screens (thin cardboard inserts) within cassettes (film holder)

  E. Naturally occurring contrast in the body

    1. Fat and air absorb little radiation
    2. Bone (calcium) absorbs more

  F. Artificial changes in contrast accomplished by ingestion or injection

    1. Gas injection

      a. Reduced density
      b. Shows outer margins of structure (e.g., pneumothorax, around lung; pneumoperitoneum, around intra-abdominal structures)
      c. Inner wall (e.g., pneumocolon)

2. Injection of iodinated contrast medium
   a. Increased density
   b. Usually within blood vessels or lymph channels
3. Ingestion of contrast medium
   a. Shows lining and lumen of structures (e.g., esophagus, stomach) by direct filling
   b. Or concentration (e.g., gallbladder)
4. Opacification of body organ system may result from excretion of medium (e.g., intravenous pyelography)

IV. Uses of diagnostic roentgenography
   A. To demonstrate presence or absence of disease processes
   B. To aid in confirming or determining diagnoses
   C. Indiscriminate use to be avoided

Throughout the practice of medicine, one of the major challenges for the physician is his ability to properly diagnose disease. Only upon the establishment of a diagnosis is treatment possible. A major key to unlocking the riddles of the disease is that of physical diagnosis. The method of examination most frequently used involves actual physical contact of the doctor with the patient and consists of auscultation, palpation, and inspection. Auscultation (listening) reveals the character of the heart sounds, the breath sounds in the lungs, and the resonance of the lungs produced by tapping the chest. Palpation shows the size and shape of various organs. Inspection demonstrates the general appearance of the patient and any visible abnormalities. By these methods the physician can detect distortions in the normal anatomy.

Diagnostic radiology provides an extension of the physical examination. It is a discipline dealing primarily with the change of visual images. By knowing the normal appearance of the various organ systems on x-ray films (roentgenograms), one can recognize variations from the normal image. Distortions shown on roentgenograms provide important clues to the nature of the abnormalities or diseases which exist. Radiology provides the only method of physical examination that enables one to see the outlines and, to some extent, the internal structures of the various organ systems in the intact individual. All other visual methods of examining these structures require removal of the covering tissues or penetration of a natural orifice by an instrument. As a consequence, there has been an increased reliance on the use of radiographs in the practice of modern medicine. Much of the basic work in developing techniques and normal standards was accomplished within the first ten years after the discovery of x-ray by Dr. Wilhelm Conrad Roentgen in 1895.

Certain limitations of the roentgenographic method must be known to the practicing physician, and some very basic visual indicators must be used in deciding whether the structures seen on the x-ray film are normal or abnormal.

It is not the purpose of this text to provide a comprehensive introduction to disease states as seen on radiographs; rather, it is to make students aware of those criteria of normality that they will be using throughout their medical careers. By the acquisition of such basic knowledge, the student should be able to profit more completely from gross anatomic observations. The fund of information available will enable him to more rapidly master sophisticated diagnostic methods by applying basic principles.

Each section of the text is introduced by an outline of the material in that section. Subsequent expansion of the outline in narrative form with illustrations and legends provides an overview of the application of diagnostic radiology.

One very basic principle which must be recognized immediately is that diagnostic radiology is the production and interpretation of a two-dimensional representation of a three-dimensional structure, using electromagnetic rays which have the potential of penetrating body tissues. The darkening of the x-ray film is caused by those x-rays which have penetrated *through* the entire body and can transmit energy to a sensitive photographic film. Anything that will prevent x-rays from passing through the body will then appear as a lighter area on the x-ray film. Objects or structures that reduce the amount of blackness of the films are called radiodensities. Those structures that allow easy transmission of the x-rays causing the film to be increasingly black are known as radiolucencies.

Within the body, various substances absorb a greater or lesser amount of x-ray, depending on the composition of the substance and the thickness of the layer of substance. Thus, calcium absorbs x-ray very effectively, leaving the film clear or white underneath the area of the organ containing the calcium, such as bone. While calcium will absorb x-rays more effectively than muscle, if a sufficient amount of muscle is interposed between the x-ray tube and the x-ray film, the amount of whiteness resulting on the film may be the same. Of the various substances normally present in the body, the following order of effectiveness of x-ray absorption should be remembered: (1) calcium, and (2) soft tissue-water density (muscle, blood, fibrous tissue, fluid), (3) fat, and (4) air (usually recognized as radiolucencies contrasted to the adjoining soft tissue densities).

More adequate studies of certain organs or organ systems can be accomplished if the natural roentgenographic density of the structure can be changed artificially. For example, on the plain film of the abdomen the roentgenographic density of the liver and the gallbladder is the same. If material of a different roentgenographic density can be made to collect within the gallbladder, then that structure can be observed separately from the density of the liver. For the organ systems that have external openings, such as the gastrointestinal system, urinary bladder, paranasal sinuses, and respiratory system, ingestion or instillation of some material may render these structures radiopaque—producing a density greater than that of the adjoining soft tissues. It is also possible in some instances to instill air into the structures; therefore, their anatomic form can be identified by an increased radiolucency. The gallbladder is a unique example in that material ingested is absorbed from the intestinal tract and concentrates within the gallbladder, permitting the demonstration of the gallbladder on the routine films. In the other organ systems that do not have external openings, change in contrast requires injection. The injection may be into the vascular system, as in angiocardiography, allowing demonstration of the internal structure of the arteries or of the veins on the roentgenograms. Placement of catheters into the venous or arterial channels enables one to selectively make radiodense those parts of the heart, arteries, or veins most necessary to study. Other substances injected into the veins may be excreted by an organ system, such as the kidneys, thereby changing the contrast of these structures and making it possible to show their form on roentgenograms. Structures within the body may also be studied by reducing the radiodensity of the surrounding structures. An example is the introduction of gas into either the pleural cavity or the peritoneal cavity. Since the gas is radiolucent, the structures outlined by the gas within the cavities may be identified as relative radiodensities. The positive contrast media (radiodense material) are usually used to show the structures within a hollow tube, such as an artery or the intestinal tract, and the radiolucent materials are used to show the appearance of the outer margins of an organ.

It is also possible to determine to some degree the ability of an organ to function. For instance, the rate and degree at which the kidneys can excrete injected contrast material is a clue to physiologic normality. Similarly, the amount of density that can be produced within the gallbladder as a result of ingestion of contrast medium demonstrates, in part, the ability of the gallbladder to concentrate bile.

Penetration of the body by the x-ray beam may be recorded on films. Most frequently, the film is placed in a Bakelite holder with a lead back. Within the holder are pieces of cardboard impregnated with a chemical. This unit is called a cassette with intensifying screens. When the x-ray beam strikes the chemical, a brief flash of light is emitted (fluorescence). The light then impinges on the x-ray film producing the image on the film. The x-ray beam may, instead, be allowed to strike a surface covered with the same chemical used in the intensifying screens. The image which is produced is then viewed directly without being recorded on a film. This process is called fluoroscopy. The image produced by the light can be intensified by optical systems or converted into electrical currents and be produced as a television image. By combining the various methods of recording, it is now possible to produce videotape of fluoroscopy or x-ray movies (cineroentgenograms). By using such techniques, one can watch the various organ systems in action. Changes in the ability of an organ system to move or change its form provide important clues in the detection of disease. Fluoroscopy and cineroentgenography allow one to follow these changes, while the usual x-ray shows the form of a given organ, such as the stomach, only at one instant of time.

Throughout the text, reference will be made to certain changes in the roentgenographic appearance of the various organ systems. These changes provide the basic parameters or indicators of normality. It is the alteration in these parameters that gives the clue to the presence of a disease state. While most of the parameters are considered separately, abnormalities are usually reflected by changes in two or more parameters. For evaluation of anatomic structure, therefore, the following characteristics should be studied: (1) density, (2) size, (3) contour, (4) location, (5) number, and (6) margination (sharpness of outline). Each of these criteria has a relatively different importance among the systems of the body. The various chapters will stress the prime indicators applicable to each organ system.

While it has not been shown that small amounts of radiation at infrequent intervals produce detectable damage to the human body, the use of radiant energy in diagnosing disease requires discrimination. The ability of the physician as a diagnostician is often reflected in the judgment he exercises in selecting the specific radiographic examination that is most likely to provide the prime clue to the diagnosis of a disease. From this standpoint, then, diagnostic radiography and radiologic interpretation must again be viewed as an expansion of the physical examination of the patient with those radiologic studies designed to explore certain anatomic areas in a way not otherwise possible.

1

CHEST

Summary of basic concepts

Chest films are the best example of naturally occurring contrast produced by varying radiation absorption. They can be separated into four main divisions: skeletal, cardiovascular, respiratory, and digestive and other mediastinal structures. The roentgenograms can be considered as a composite of these different organ systems, but organ systems are evaluated independently in chest films.

I. Skeletal system
  A. Components
    1. Clavicles
    2. Scapulae
    3. Ribs
    4. Thoracic spine
    5. Portions of cervical and lumbar spine
    6. Shoulder joints
    7. Sternum
  B. Roentgenographic parameters
    1. Number
    2. Density
    3. Contour
    4. Location (alignment)
    5. Size
  C. Common roentgenographic positions
    1. Ribs—part of ribs to be studied to be closest to film
      a. P-A (posteroanterior)
      b. A-P (anteroposterior)
      c. Obliques
    2. Sternum
      a. P-A
      b. Lateral
    3. Thoracic spine
      a. A-P
      b. Lateral
  D. Application
    1. May reflect systemic or focal disease (e.g., sternum in arthritis)
    2. Location indicator of volume of heart or lungs
    3. Osseous structure shaped by adjoining structures, particularly pulsating columns, as aorta
    4. Cartilage usually nonopaque (radiolucent) and nondemonstrable

II. Cardiovascular system
  A. Components
      1. Heart
      2. Aorta
      3. Subclavian arteries
      4. Innominate artery
      5. Pulmonary arteries
      6. Pulmonary veins
      7. Vena cava
  B. Roentgenographic parameters
      1. Size—relative (related to chest size) or absolute (beyond normal measurements)
      2. Contour
      3. Density
      4. Function
      5. Location
  C. Heart
      1. Size
          a. Increased
              (1) Dilatation (Most common—slight contour change)
                  (a) Intrinsic (wall weakened)
                  (b) Extrinsic (increased volume, e.g. pericardial effusion)
              (2) Hypertrophy (Less enlargement—more contour change)
          b. Decreased (e.g., blood volume reduction)
          c. Roentgenographic cardiac outline: epipericardial and pericardial tissue included
      2. Contour—chamber disproportion
          a. Left ventricular enlargement
              (1) Apex rounded—projects downward
              (2) Cardiac apex behind inferior vena cava and esophagus (lateral view)
          b. Right ventricular enlargement
              (1) Fullness anterior portion heart
              (2) Heart displaced from pressure against sternum
          c. Left atrial enlargement
              (1) Displacement adjoining structures—esophagus, lung, bronchi
              (2) Veins from right lung received to right of midline—right lung distorted by atrial enlargement
          d. Right atrial enlargement
              (1) Most difficult chamber to evaluate
              (2) Fills in retrosternal space
      3. Density
          a. Increased
              (1) Natural—calcification
              (2) Artificial (iodides)—for chamber size and pathway of blood flow
          b. Decreased—all artificial—gas injection (carbon dioxide)
      4. Function
          a. Methods
              (1) Fluoroscopy
              (2) Cineroentgenography
              (3) Videotape
              (4) Plain films or angiocardiography

      b. Parameters—pulsations: key to status myocardium and pericardium
        (1) Rhythm
        (2) Rate
        (3) Amplitude
      c. Points of opposite pulsation: edges of individual chambers
    5. Common projection used (specific chambers brought into profile)
      a. P-A   d. Right oblique
      b. A-P   e. Left oblique
      c. Lateral
    6. Distortion of surrounding structures by cardiac abnormalities
      a. Air-containing lung displaced and compressed: total or focal cardiac enlargement
      b. Barium filled esophagus: by cardiac or aortic enlargement
D. Pulmonary vessels
    1. Enlarged
      a. Excess volume of blood—shunt—arteries and/or veins
      b. Stasis
        (1) Increased resistance—peripheral or central arteries and/or veins
        (2) Decreased rate of return of blood to heart—veins
    2. Small
      a. Stenosis pulmonary arterial circuit—arteries and/or veins
      b. Pulmonary hypertension—veins
    3. Unusual location or contour—anomalous formation
E. Superior and inferior vena cavae
    1. Enlarged
      a. Obstruction
        (1) Intracardiac—decompensation
        (2) Extracardiac—tumor pressure
      b. Excess blood volume—anomalous veins
    2. Small—compressed by adjoining tissue
F. Aorta and great vessels
    1. Size
      a. Enlarged—displace adjoining structures (e.g., trachea and esophagus)
        (1) Wall weakened (e.g., senility, infection)
        (2) Increased pressure (e.g., hypertension, aortic insufficiency)
        (3) Increased flow (e.g., extracardiac shunt)
      b. Small
        (1) Decreased volume (e.g., intracardiac shunt)
        (2) Reduced thrust (e.g., aortic stenosis)
    2. Contour
      a. Tortuous (e.g., senility)
      b. Irregular (e.g., aneurysm)
    3. Density—increased
      a. Physiologic calcification
      b. Artificial (iodide injection)
    4. Location—aorta
      a. Left—usual
      b. Right—congenital anomaly

III. Respiratory system
   A. Components
      1. Lungs
      2. Pleura
      3. Hila
   B. Lung
      1. Segmentation
         a. Right lung
            (1) Upper lobe: apical, posterior and anterior segments
            (2) Middle lobe: lateral and medial segments
            (3) Lower lobe: superior, posterior basal, lateral basal, anterior basal, and medial basal segments
         b. Left lung
            (1) Upper lobe
               (a) Apical-posterior and anterior segments
               (b) Lingula: superior and inferior segments
            (2) Lower lobe: superior, posterior basal, lateral basal, anterior-medial basal segments
         c. Accessory lobes—portions of other lobes set off by pleural reflection
            (1) Azygos lobe
            (2) Inferior medial segment right lower lobe
      2. Size
         a. Decrease—pulmonary vessels and bronchi crowded
            (1) Collapse
               (a) Obstruction   (b) Contraction
            (2) Compression—extrinsic pressure
         b. Increase—pulmonary vessels and bronchi spread
            (1) Overexpansion
               (a) Compensatory overexpansion
               (b) Emphysema
            (2) Athlete's lung
      3. Density
         a. Increased—loss of air
            (1) Atelectasis
            (2) Consolidation—fluid
            (3) Abnormal tissue (e.g., tumor)
            (4) Configuration clue to etiology
               (a) Wedge-shaped—atelectasis, infarct
               (b) Spherical, lobulated with or without calcification—tumor or granuloma
         b. Decreased—excess air
            (1) Increased volume
               (a) Focal
               (b) General
            (2) Emphysematous bullae
         c. Artificial density increase
            (1) Trachea and bronchi (bronchogram)
            (2) Vascular injection

C. Pleura or hila
1. Density and size—increased
   a. Scarring
   b. Soft tissues and/or calcification
   c. Tumor
2. Location
   a. Position of hila proportionate to lung expansion
   b. Level of hila indicator of volume change of lung segments
   c. Level of fissures also indicator of change in volume of lung

IV. Digestive system and mediastinal structures
A. Esophagus
1. Examination requires change in density—usually barium but catheter or air may be used
2. Normally seen only partially due to peristalsis but if abnormal may show in entirety
3. Adequate evaluation requires study of function by fluoroscopy with or without cineroentgenography
4. Effect of adjoining abnormalities
   a. Displace
   b. Deform
   c. Obstruct (causing dilatation or delay in emptying)
5. Intrinsic disease
   a. Irregularity of lumen   c. Spasm
   b. Abnormal contraction   d. Decreased motility (function)
6. Debility or morbid physical status of individual may decrease potential for function

B. Other mediastinal structures—thymus, lymph nodes, and neurofibrous tissues
1. Changes in size
   a. Enlargement may obscure adjoining structures by displacing lung
   b. Location of mass key to nature of lesion
      (1) Anterior—thymus, nodes
      (2) Posterior—neurogenic or fibrous in origin
2. Contour
   a. Lobulation
      (1) Multiple masses
      (2) Peritracheal lymph nodes
      (3) Lobulated thymus
   b. Smooth margination
      (1) Primary tumor
      (2) Cyst
      (3) Vascular
3. Density
   a. Increased—calcification
      (1) Lymph nodes   (3) Dermoid cyst
      (2) Teratoma   (4) Angioma
   b. Decreased—fat or air
      (1) Lipoma
      (2) Emphysema

The basic principles of radiography using naturally occurring differences in radiation absorption to define anatomic structures can now be applied. The chest, with calcium in the skeletal system, air in the lung, fat in the subcutaneous tissues and between the muscle bundles, and soft tissue densities of the heart, mediastinum, and muscles of the thoracic wall, illustrates all of the various absorbing abilities of the tissues of the body (Figs. 1-1 and 1-2).

It has been emphasized that any radiograph is a two-dimensional depiction of a three-dimensional structure. One must also remember that this is a method of physically examining a patient. The x-ray films may be viewed system by system. Four major systems are well demonstrated on the film of the chest. These include the skeletal system, respiratory system, cardiovascular system, and di-

Text continued on p. 19.

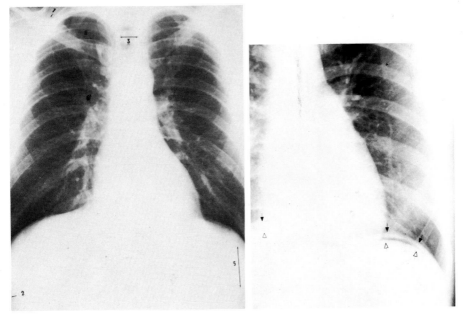

Fig. 1-1   Fig. 1-2

Fig. 1-1. P-A chest, normal. Contrasting radiodensities of soft tissue, fat, calcium, and air outline anatomic structures. The edge of the skin (companion shadow clavicle—*1*) contrasts against the air. Radiolucent fat is present in the supraclavicular area and between the liver edge and the abdominal musculature (*2*). The air in the trachea (*3*) shows its diameter. The density of the cervical muscles (*4*) is the same as that of the spleen (*5*), with the only difference being the difference in size of the relative organs. Pleura, when surrounded by air, is visible. An unusual slip of pleura is seen in the right upper lung (*6*), representing an azygos lobe with the density of the azygos vein hidden behind the medial aspect of the right clavicle. The cortical margins of the ribs are denser than the central area; this is an indication of the amount of calcium per cubic millimeter of tissue.

Fig. 1-2. There has been a change in the roentgenographic density of the tissues beneath the diaphragmatic leaves, with free air within the abdominal cavity. The arrows show the thickness of the diaphragmatic leaf and the inferior margin of the intra-abdominal gas from abdominal surgery.

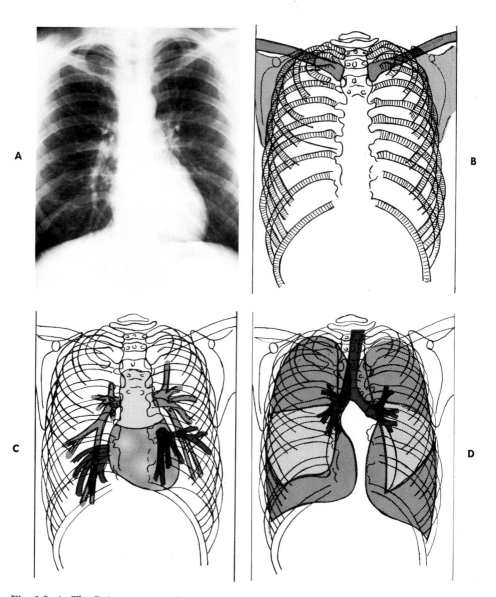

Fig. 1-3. A, The P-A projection of the chest shows the overlap of the various organ systems. The line drawings show the relationship of the osseous (**B**), cardiovascular (**C**), and respiratory (**D**) structures. The major anatomic structures are detectable. Identify pulmonary vessels and veins, the major bronchi, and the diagrammed portions of the osseous system. The position of the hila is normal, with the left lying somewhat higher than the right. The sharp demarcation of the cardiac margin shows that there is aerated lung surrounding the heart.

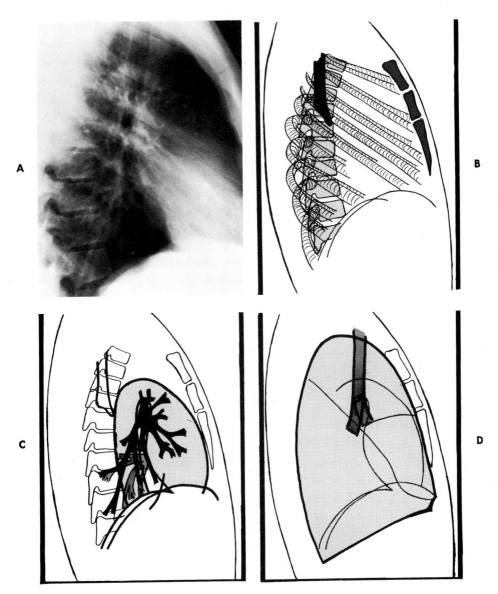

Fig. 1-4. A, The lateral view of the chest superimposes right- and left-sided structures but more clearly defines other areas. The trachea, the retrosternal area, and the retrocardiac area are all seen. The overlapping of the anatomic systems can be appreciated from the diagrams.

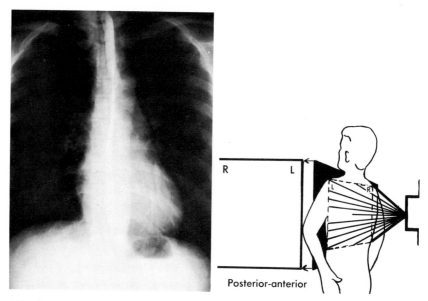

Fig. 1-5. The P-A projection. The aortic arch is the most superior prominence projecting to the left causing minor pressure on the esophagus. Next inferiorly is the prominence of the main pulmonary artery, overlying the left mainstem bronchus. Below the mainstem bronchus is the left auricular appendage. The rounded lower border of the heart is the margin of the left ventricle. The right atrium projects to the right of the mediastinum.

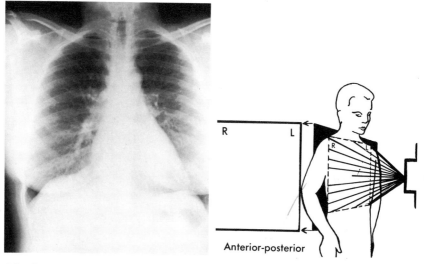

Fig. 1-6. The A-P projection resembles the P-A.

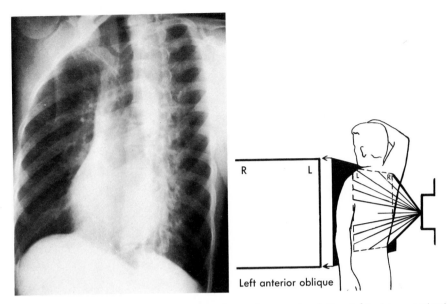

Fig. 1-7. The left anterior oblique projection shows the margin of the right atrium projecting to the patient's right anteriorly and the left ventricle projecting posteriorly and to the patient's left. The junction of the right and left ventricles lies just above the junction of the left hemidiaphragm and the cardiac outline. The ascending aorta lies superiorly on the patient's right. The arc of the descending aorta can be seen overlying the spine.

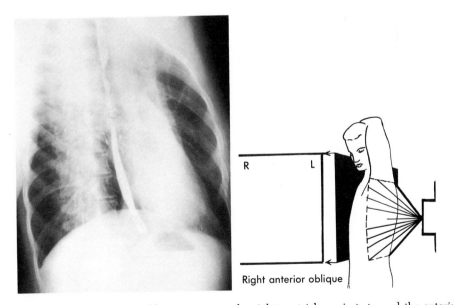

Fig. 1-8. In the right anterior oblique projection the right ventricle projects toward the anterior left lateral aspect of the patient's chest; the prominence superior to the ventricle represents the pulmonary artery. The left atrium lies against the anterior aspect of the barium filled esophagus; the aortic arch produces a notch on the esophagus superiorly.

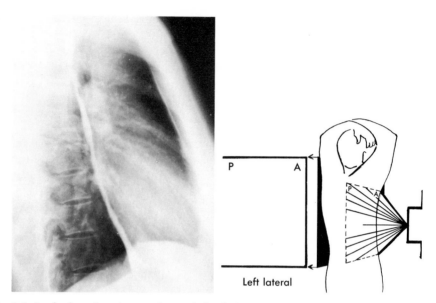

Fig. 1-9. In the lateral projection the air behind the sternum contrasts against the pulmonary artery; the right ventricle lies in apposition to the posterior aspect of the sternum inferiorly. Posteriorly, the left atrium causes pressure on the descending esophagus.

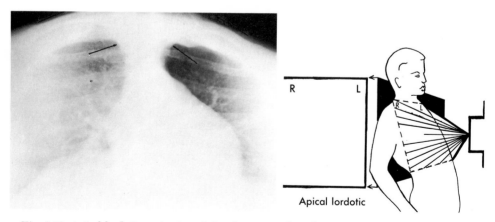

Fig. 1-10. Apical lordotic projection of the chest is used to show the areas normally hidden behind the upper rib cage and overlying scapulas. The clavicles lie above the rib cage. The difference in the density of the right upper lobe and left upper lobe is the result of overlying breast tissue. The heart appears unusual as a result of the axis of projection. The brachiocephalic vessels (solid arrows) are brought into prominence.

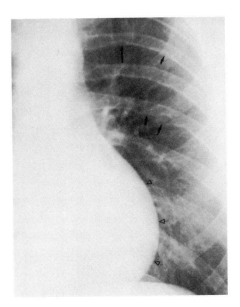

Fig 1-11. Abnormalities of the osseous system may relate to abnormalities of the cardiovascular system. The left ventricle is quite rounded (open arrows). In addition, inferior margins of the ribs show irregular indentations (scalloping—solid arrows). This represents the result of dilated collateral circulation as the result of coarctation of the aorta.

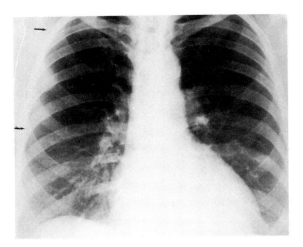

Fig. 1-12. A change in density by a soft tissue mass is identified. This is a hemispheric density with its flat surface against the pleura. It lies somewhere between the solid arrows, and its margins can be identified clearly. This could arise from the pleura, intercostal vessels, or ribs. It is in actuality a neurinoma originating from the intercostal nerve.

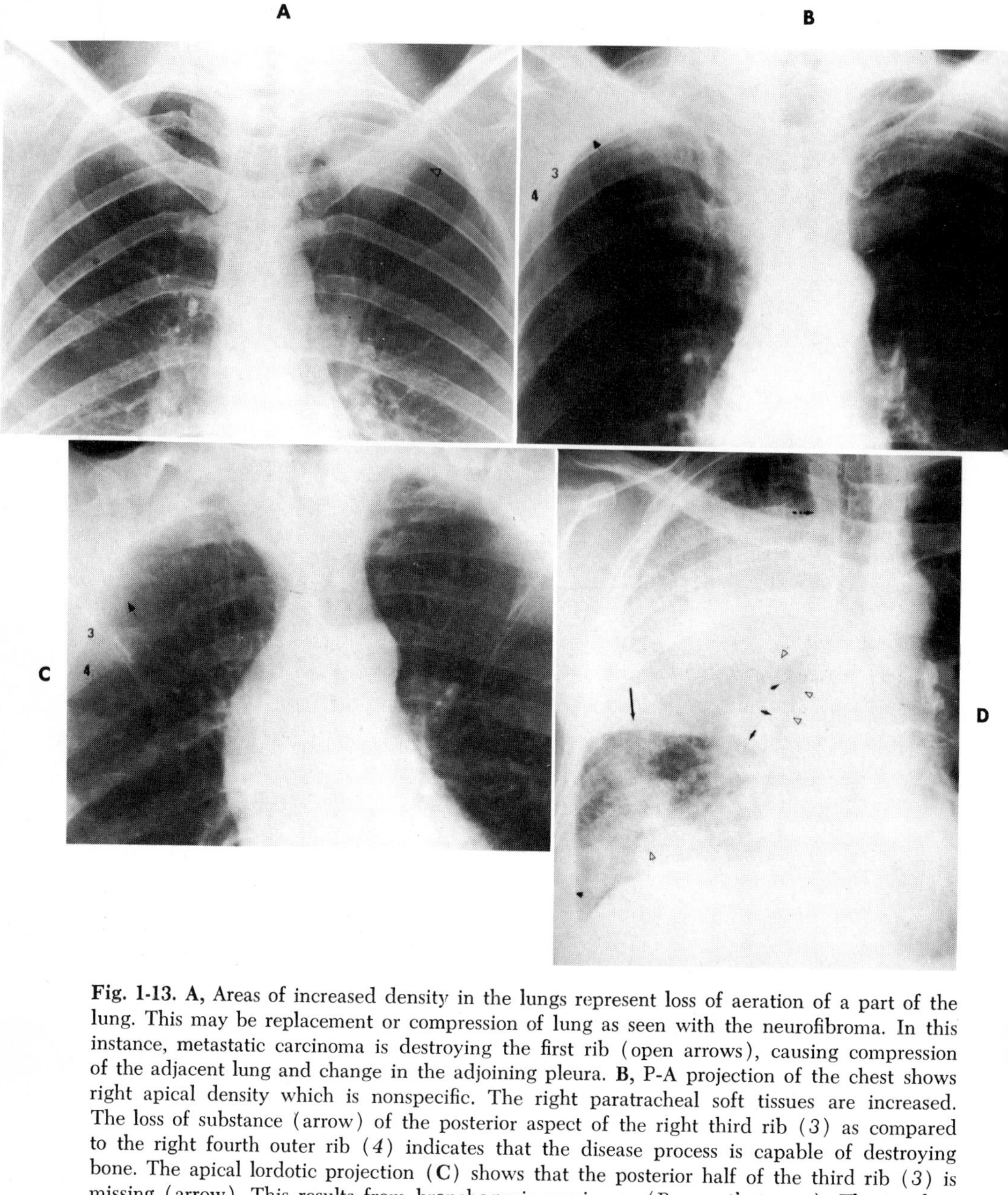

Fig. 1-13. A, Areas of increased density in the lungs represent loss of aeration of a part of the lung. This may be replacement or compression of lung as seen with the neurofibroma. In this instance, metastatic carcinoma is destroying the first rib (open arrows), causing compression of the adjacent lung and change in the adjoining pleura. **B,** P-A projection of the chest shows right apical density which is nonspecific. The right paratracheal soft tissues are increased. The loss of substance (arrow) of the posterior aspect of the right third rib (3) as compared to the right fourth outer rib (4) indicates that the disease process is capable of destroying bone. The apical lordotic projection (**C**) shows that the posterior half of the third rib (3) is missing (arrow). This results from bronchogenic carcinoma (Pancoast's tumor). The involvement of the pleura, lung, and rib indicates the malignant nature of the disease. **D,** Evaluation of the abnormalities seen on the P-A chest roentgenogram may provide answers to many questions. A tumor mass in the region of the right hilum is projecting into the bronchus in the right lower lobe (short solid arrows) with its inferior margin outlined by the adjoining aerated lung. This has produced compression and angulation of the bronchi (upper open arrows). The air bronchogram in the lower lobes (lower open arrow) shows that the alveoli are fllled with fluid. The separation of the lower lobe from the rib cage (short solid arrow) shows the amount of fluid present in the pleural space. The long solid arrow shows consolidation in the anterior portion of the right upper lobe producing the solid white area. The superior mediastinum (dotted arrow) is wide, showing involvement by tumor.

gestive system (Figs. 1-3 and 1-4). A mental check-off list, system by system, will ensure that each of these systems has been evaluated on a chest film (Fig. 1-5 to Fig. 1-10). Studies have indicated that a radiologist initially views a chest film, rapidly scans the film and more intensely studies any one area that catches his attention. This is acceptable for the experienced physician, but during the learning phase, it is better to use careful systematic evaluation of the anatomic structures.

Use of radiographic studies also allows detection of interdependent abnormalities. For instance, diseases of the cardiovascular system may suggest that the skeletal system is also involved. An example of this would be the cardiac and aortic changes consistent with coarctation of the aorta. Notching of the ribs provides substantiating evidence (Fig. 1-11). The same line of reasoning may be applied to the respiratory system, wherein a nodular density in the lung (Fig. 1-12) may be nonspecific; however, if there is destruction of one of the ribs on the opposite side, the diagnosis would be neoplasm, most likely metastatic (Fig. 1-13).

Skeletal system

For study of the skeletal system on the routine films of the chest, both a posteroanterior (P-A) and a lateral film are required as a minimum. It is often surprising to realize how many skeletal structures are identifiable on the chest films. Those structures that are obvious and should be studied routinely include: (1) clavicles, (2) ribs, (3) scapulae, (4) thoracic spine, (5) manubrium, (6) sternum. In addition, other osseous structures are shown although not as well as those mentioned, but with sufficient clarity that abnormalities can be found. These would include: (1) the lower cervical spine, particularly in the posteroanterior (P-A) projection of the chest; (2) the upper lumbar spine in both the P-A and the lateral projections; (3) the shoulder joints; (4) acromioclavicular joints, and (5) head of the humeri, including the bicipital grooves. It is a common occurrence to make the roentgenographic diagnosis of calcific peritendonitis of one shoulder on a routine roentgenographic study of the chest.

Changes suggesting abnormalities

Abnormalities of the osseosus structures may be reflected in various ways.

Density. Change in the density, either generally or focally, is the most common criterion used for the detection of disease. Demineralization of the skeletal system as a whole is reflected early in the thoracic spine and the ribs. If demineralization is generalized, osteoporosis or osteomalacia should be considered. Osteoporosis of old age is by far the most frequent cause of this loss of calcium. Focal loss of radiodensity would most likely represent a neoplastic disease, although infectious processes and healing fractures can also cause such a change. The amount of calcium in the bones may be increased above the normal level. Osteoblastic metastasis, systemic metabolic disturbance causing excessive calcification, and toxic agents such as fluorine, all may produce bone density greater

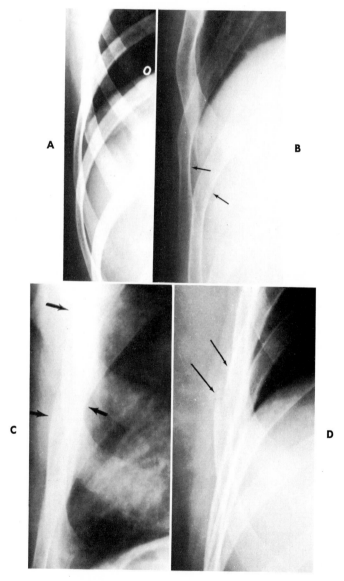

Fig. 1-14. Variation in density and appearance of the osseous system seen on chest roentgeno-grams reflects the general bodily status. The ribs in **A** are normal; in **B** they are osteoporotic, with thin cortices and poor calcium content; in **C** metastatic disease of prostate has produced diffuse increased density and loss of cortical definition; in **D** there are two acute fractures in osteoporotic ribs (arrows).

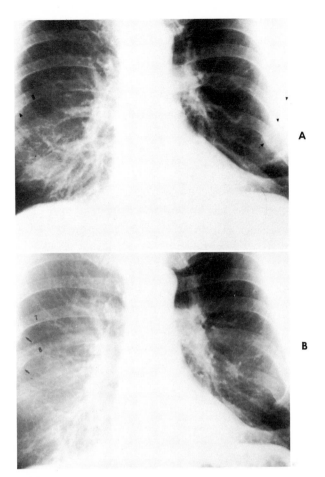

Fig. 1-15. A, Rib fractures may be difficult to identify. An acute fracture of the eighth rib on the right (solid arrow) is seen on the original study, as are old healed rib fractures on the left. **B,** The film taken 3 years later shows healing of the fracture of the eighth rib and in addition healing of the fracture of the seventh rib which was present before but undetected. The multiplicity of fractures in this case resulted from coughing, but other injury would indicate that there is lack of part of the bone, probably as the result of osteoporosis.

than normal. Determination of increased density is somewhat more difficult than that of reduced density since, in the young adult, the bones may normally be fairly heavy and appear very white on the films (Figs. 1-14 and 1-15).

Contour. Irregularity of the outline of bone may be developmental, since bone sometimes records stress experienced during the time of development. Even after maturation the contour of the bones, particularly of the vertebral bodies, is sometimes altered by unusual stress. Bone continues to remodel throughout life. The osseous structures may also show pressure from adjoining organs, particularly if the adjoining structure is pulsatile. An example of this is erosion of the thoracic vertebrae by aortic aneurysm (Figs. 1-16 and 1-17). The sternum may bow rather sharply anteriorly if the heart, particularly the right ventricle,

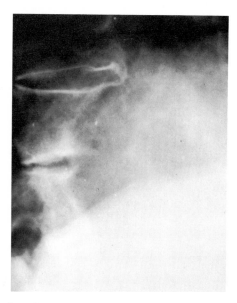

Fig. 1-16. Erosion of the low thoracic vertebrae by aneurysm of the aorta leaves the adjoining intervertebral discs partially intact. The resiliency of the disc makes it less susceptible to the pulsating column of blood in the dilated aorta. Cardiovascular disease thereby affects the osseous system.

is enlarged. Classically, notching of the ribs is produced by dilated intercostal vessels. This condition was initially described in coarctation of the aorta; however, any pathologic process which causes an increased runoff of the blood through the venous system or an excessive demand on the arterial system may produce similar changes.

Alignment. Since bone is deposited under stress, alteration in alignment may change both the density and the contour. For example, along the concavity of a scoliosis, the vertebrae become narrow in their vertical dimension and may show increased density. The ribs also have an expected alignment, even though the bony structures are not in direct apposition. Thus, decreased distance between the ribs on one side of the chest compared with the other side may result from: (1) scoliosis, (2) atelectasis of the lung, (3) muscle spasm with splinting, and (4) intrinsic derangement of the bony structures posteriorly at the costovertebral articulations (Fig. 1-18).

Size. Any systemic stimulus to bone formation is reflected in the osseous structures of the chest. One example is the increased anteroposterior diameter of the low thoracic vertebrae in acromegaly (Fig. 1-19). The most frequent cause of the increase in size is hypertrophic response of old age; this condition is seen most frequently about the spine, but is also noticeable about the rib ends. While focal gigantism may occur in the extremities, it is much less common in the structures of the chest. Diminution in size of the vertebrae or the ribs may result from either erosion or failure of development. Poor muscular development resulting

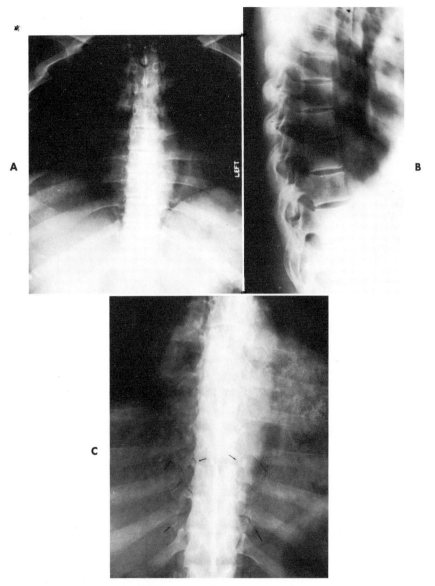

Fig. 1-17. The normal thoracic spine contrasts with the spine in Fig. 1-16. **A,** The form of the vertebral bodies, the density of the vertebral bodies, and the relative cortical thickness are normal. **B,** In the lateral projection the small solid arrow shows early hypertrophic degenerative change, not remarkable for a 37-year-old. **C,** The costovertebral articulations (central arrows) bridge the intervertebral discs; the articulations between the transverse processes and the tubercles of the ribs (lateral arrows) are thrown open by this view taken with the beam angled toward the head.

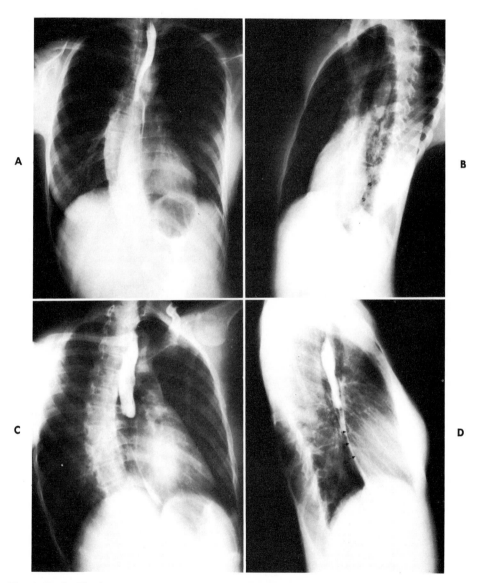

Fig. 1-18. A, The heart appears peculiar on the roentgenographs because of the scoliosis of the thoracic spine curving to the right. **B,** The posterior border of the left ventricle (open arrows), as seen in the left anterior oblique projection, appears somewhat prominent because of some rotation of the heart. **C,** The cardiac structures appear relatively normal in the right anterior oblique projection. **D,** The left atrium (solid arrows) and left ventricle (open arrow), as seen in the lateral projection, lie somewhat posteriorly because of the scoliosis. Such deformity occasionally produces hemic murmurs.

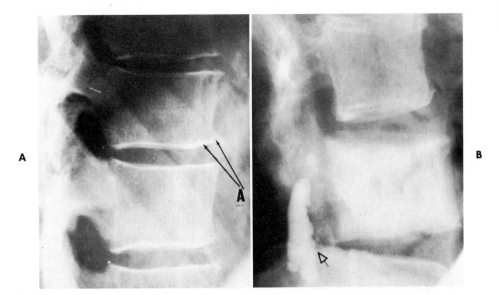

Fig. 1-19. A, Systemic disease may manifest itself in the thoracic vertebrae. Excess bone deposited on the anterior margin of the thoracolumbar vertebrae is characteristic of acromegaly. The new bone formation (*A*) lies between the posteriorly pointing arrow, which indicates the original cortex, and a more anteriorly placed arrow, which locates the new cortex. Notice that the central lucency in the body (Hans cleft) is not present in the new bone. **B,** This also shows an enlargement of the vertebrae by disposition of unusual bone from Paget's disease. The bony proliferation is around the margins of the vertebrae with a coarse trabecular pattern. The pedicles and the posterior elements of the vertebrae as well as the bodies are involved.

from either paralysis or abnormalities which prevent motion causes the involved bones to be smaller.

Number. In the chest, variation in the number of bony structures is probably the most frequent anomaly. This anomaly is represented by either a rudimentary or absent twelfth rib or the presence of a cervical rib. It is quite common to find thirteen ribs on one side with twelve on the other, or eleven ribs on one side and twelve on the other. Fusion of adjoining bony structures such as the vertebrae or the ribs may reduce the number of structures. Such anomalies, however, are very easily identified since the resultant combined structure is much larger than that normally expected. On occasions, however, a rib or a vertebra may be completely missing as the result of either surgical intervention or some destructive disease, such as infection or tumor. It is very easy in these cases to overlook the abnormality unless special care is devoted to the study of the skeletal system.

Projections used

While in most instances the use of the P-A and lateral projections of the chest is quite adequate for a satisfactory view of the bony structures of the thorax, special films of the ribs should be used in all instances when a fracture is suspected. Specific films of the shoulders, clavicle, and sternum are used to determine more clearly the internal structure of these bones. It is important to remember that the bone closest to the film at the time of exposure will have the sharpest definition. For this purpose, if the anterior part of the rib or sternum is to be radiographed, the beam should enter through the back of the patient, and the part to be examined should be against the film.

Cardiovascular system

While the cardiovascular system should actually be considered as a single system, the individual components may be isolatedly affected by disease. Inter-relationships between the various components, therefore, should be considered in assessment of disease processes and also in relation to the normal appearance. Structures that comprise this system are: heart, aorta, subclavian arteries, innominate artery, pulmonary arteries, pulmonary veins, and superior and inferior vena cavae. These structures, if looked for, can be identified routinely on P-A and lateral projections of the chest. Other vascular structures may be seen occasionally but are not always identifiable on routine chest films. These structures include the azygos vein, intercostal arteries, internal mammary arteries, carotid arteries, abdominal aorta in its upper portion, and bronchial arteries.

HEART

The heart produces the largest radiopacity within the thoracic cage, and the viewer almost automatically looks at this area first (Figs. 1-20 to 1-22).

Changes suggesting abnormalities

Size. Variations in the size of the heart produce one of the major difficulties in diagnostic roentgenographic examinations of the chest because so many factors may alter the apparent size of the heart without appreciably affecting the true size of the heart. The illustrations of the apparent cardiac size difference between expiration and inspiration show the most common cause of variation in apparent heart size (Fig. 1-23). It cannot be overstressed that the heart is a three-dimensional structure and, therefore, requires evaluation not only in its transverse diameter, as demonstrated on the P-A projection, but also in its anteroposterior diameter, as shown on the lateral projection. Failure to be familiar with the lateral projection is one of the most frequent weak points in students' use of roentgenographic examinations of the chest. One may say, then, that volume change is apparent or real, depending upon the relative position of the heart within the thoracic cage. The heart may be relatively enlarged, that is, apparently large as compared to the overall size of the thoracic cage, or it may be absolutely enlarged, that is, greater than the predicted normal measurement of any of the axes of the heart. Chest deformity may also cause apparent cardiac abnormality (Fig. 1-24). It must be remembered that the heart is recorded at only one interval of time and is subject to diastolic–systolic variation, and, to a certain extent, variation in the projection utilized. For example, an adult heart placed in a child's chest would be both relatively and absolutely increased in volume. On the other hand, a normal heart of an obese patient placed in the chest of a similarly statured

Text continued on p. 32.

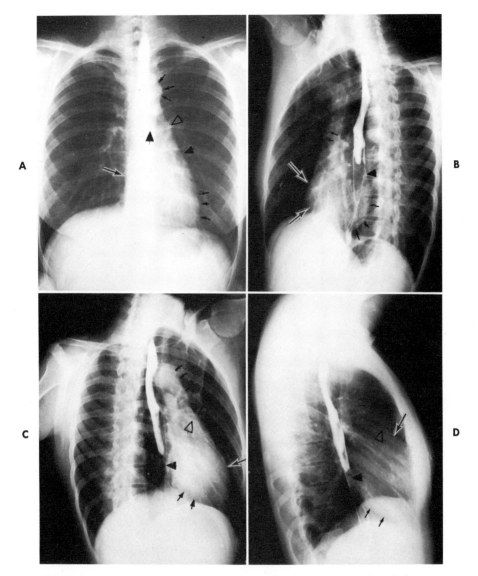

Fig. 1-20. The normal appearance of the heart. **A,** In the P-A projection the solid arrows outline the aorta and left ventricle, and the long solid arrow, the region of the right atrium. The
pulmonary artery (open arrow), and left atrial appendage (broad-tailless arrow) are identifiable along the left cardiac margin. The left mainstem bronchus (broad-tailed arrow) lies immediately above the left atrium. The same structures are identified by similar arrows in the
following illustrations. **B,** In the left anterior oblique projection, the left ventricle is now seen
to project posteriorly (solid arrows). **C,** The right anterior oblique projection shows the
aorta projecting superiorly and anteriorly and the left ventricle projecting inferiorly and posteriorly. **D,** The lateral projection shows the right ventricle in the retrosternal clear space. The
tailless arrow indicates the area of the left atrium projecting against the esophagus. The left
ventricle (lower solid arrows) is the posterior inferior chamber, separated from the diaphragmatic surface by the aerated lung.

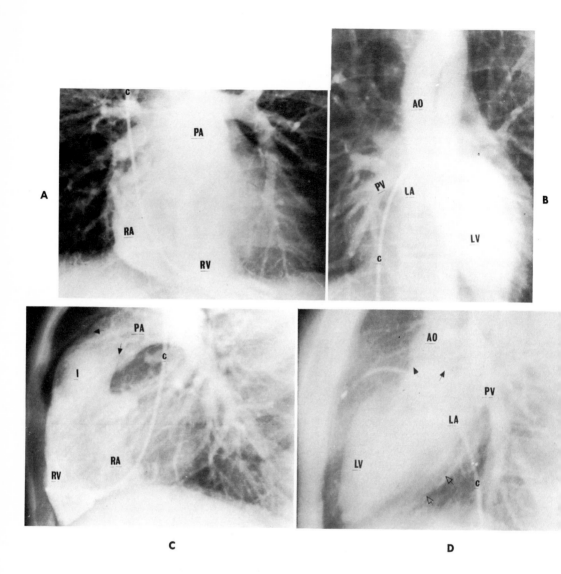

Fig. 1-21. Injection of contrast medium (angiocardiography) changes the density of the chambers of the heart. **A,** Introduction of a catheter (*c*) into the right ventricle produces an outline of the right atrium (*RA*), right ventricle (*RV*), and main pulmonary artery (*PA*). This is the view as seen in the A-P projection. These are the normal relationships of the right-sided chambers. **B,** Delayed A-P film shows the return of the contrast medium to the heart through the pulmonary veins (*PV*). The left atrium (*LA*) is opacified and the left ventricle (*LV*) outlined. The aorta (*AO*) is dense showing its ascending, horizontal, and descending portions. **C,** The lateral projection shows the relationship of the right atrium (*RA*), right ventricle (*RV*), the infundibulum of the right ventricle (*I*), the pulmonary valves (solid arrows), and the undivided segment of the pulmonary artery (*PA*). The peripheral arterial tree is opacified. **D,** The left chambers of the heart, as seen in the lateral projection. The left atrium (*LA*) and left ventricle (*LV*) are opacified. The aorta (*AO*), seen in profile, rises superiorly out of the heart, with the aortic valves (solid arrows) causing indentation in the column. The pulmonary veins are still opacified (*PV*). The distance between the opacified lumen of the left ventricle and the outer wall (open arrows) shows the thickness of the wall.

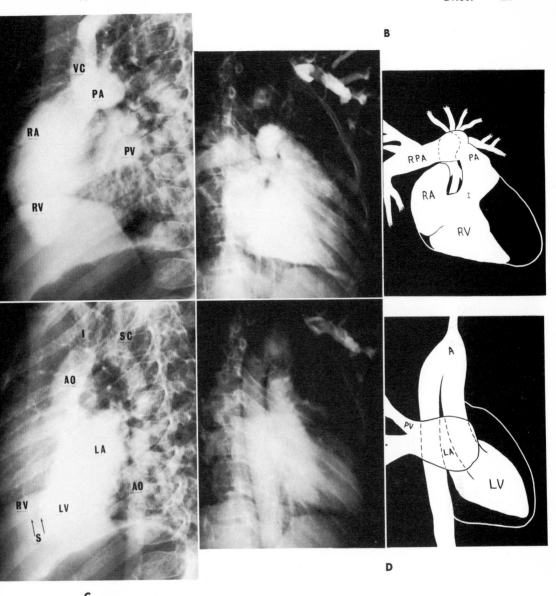

Fig. 1-22. A, The left anterior oblique projection. The relative location of the vena cava (*VC*), right atrium (*RA*), and right ventricle (*RV*) are seen. The pulmonary veins (*PV*) are already beginning to opacify. **B,** The right anterior oblique projection shows the right ventricle (*RV*) and infundibulum (*I*) to lie somewhat anteriorly, feeding to the pulmonary artery (*PA*) above the pulmonary valves. The right atrium (*RA*) is partially superimposed upon the right pulmonary artery (*RPA*). **C,** The left anterior oblique projection shows opacification of the left atrium (*LA*) and left ventricle (*LV*) with the margin of the right ventricle in apposition to the opacified left ventricle. The arrows and S indicate the level of the ventricular septum. The aorta (*AO*) rises up and out of the heart mass and gives off the innominate artery (*I*) and the subclavian artery on the left (*SC*). **D,** Opacification of the left side of the heart shows the left ventricle (*LV*) lies inferiorly and posteriorly and the left atrium (*LA*) projects posteriorly. The aorta is seen head on (*A*). (Reprinted by permission from Abrams, H. L.: Angiocardiographic interpretation in congenital heart disease, Springfield, Ill., 1956, Charles C Thomas.

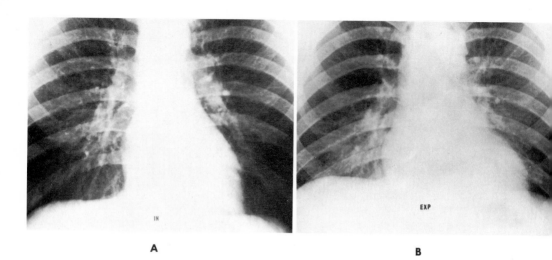

A   B

Fig. 1-23. A plain film of the chest may, as a result of poor inspiratory effort, appear to show cardiac enlargement. **A,** With deep inspiration, the heart appears normal in diameter and the superior mediastinum is also normal. **B,** With expiration, the heart appears broad and the superior mediastinum appears wide.

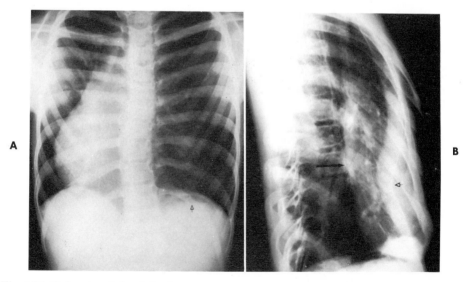

Fig. 1-24. Deformity of the skeletal system may produce severe distortion of the cardiac structures. **A,** The heart lies in the right side of the chest. The left side of the chest is identifiable by the gas bubble of the stomach (open arrow). While this would appear to be a severe cardiac abnormality, the lateral projection (**B**) shows a very narrow A-P diameter of the chest resulting from the severe retraction of the sternum (open arrow) and an anterior curve of the thoracic spine (lordosis) instead of the usual kyphosis (solid arrow). The resultant deformity of the chest has produced displacement of the heart to the right and may produce hemic murmurs.

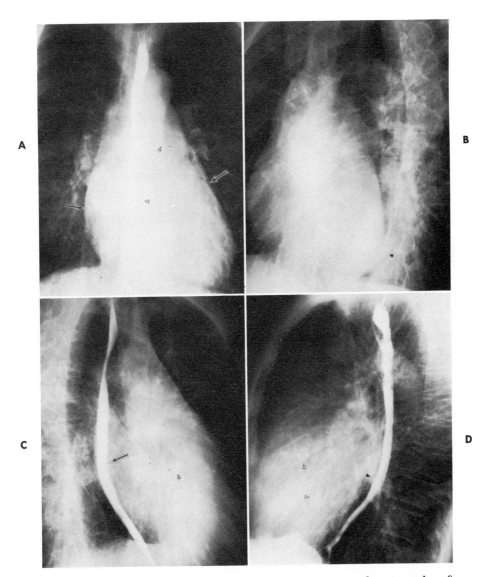

Fig. 1-25. True cardiac abnormalities may be reflected by change in cardiac size and configuration. This heart is enlarged. **A,** The P-A projection shows prominence of the left auricular appendage (white arrow) and the left mainstem bronchus lies somewhat high (upper open arrow). A double density (left atrium) extends to the right of the heart (solid arrow). The esophagus is deviated to the right by the left atrium (lower open arrow). **B,** In the left anterior oblique position, the left ventricular tip lies very low and is posteriorly placed (solid arrow). This indicates left ventricular enlargement. **C,** In the right anterior oblique projection, the barium filled esophagus shows impression on its anterior margins by the enlarged left atrium (solid arrow). Calcification is observed in the region of the aortic valve (open arrow). **D,** The lateral projection shows the calcification of the aortic valve (upper open arrow) and calcification in the region of the mitral valve (lower open arrow). The esophagus is displaced posteriorly (solid arrow) by the enlarged left atrium. These findings are characteristic of mitral and aortic valvular stenosis, in this instance, a result of rheumatic fever.

asthenic individual, while still measuring within normal limits on its various axes, would be relatively increased in comparison to the shape and size of the chest.

Enlargement of the heart usually reflects dilatation of the heart rather than hypertrophy. Hypertrophy may well produce alteration in contour; however, it is dilatation that produces the enlargement seen on roentgenograms of the chest. Causes of dilatation may be either intrinsic—weakening of the wall, which allows the heart to "balloon"—or extrinsic—increased blood volume being forced into the heart. The usual cause of such an increase in blood volume is lack of protection of the individual chambers by incompetent valves, as in aortic insufficiency (Figs. 1-25 and 1-26). Hypertrophy of the heart muscle produces less overall enlargement.

The heart may, on occasions, appear small. An overexpanded chest resulting from emphysema may make the heart seem small. Cardiac size is usually estimated by visually integrating the relative size of the chest, the apparent size of the heart in all dimensions, the level of the diaphragmatic leaves, and the habitus of the individual being examined. To gain facility in making intelligent evaluation, one must study a large number of various chest roentgenographic examinations to become familiar with the normal variation (Figs. 1-27 to 1-34).

Contour. While the overall size of the heart is indicative of the total cardiac status and the amount of work required of the heart, the configuration of the heart is the roentgenologic indicator of the relative size of the individual cham-

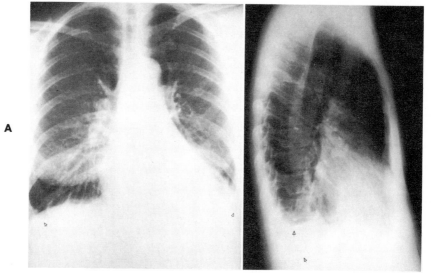

A   B

Fig. 1-26. The heart is enlarged in both the P-A (**A**) and lateral (**B**) projections. There is loss of aeration of the posterior costophrenic sulci as the result of pleural fluid (open arrows). The pulmonary vessels are engorged, indicative of cardiac failure. This patient has a long history of high blood pressure as a result of kidney disease. The pleural and pulmonary changes are the result of underlying cardiovascular disease.

bers. One must, therefore, be aware of the relative location of the chambers. On the superior posterior margin of the heart lies the left atrium; inferiorly lies the left ventricle; on the anterior margin lies the right ventricle. As the heart is viewed in the lateral projection, the tip of the right atrium also comprises a portion of the anterior superior cardiac margin. As it is viewed in the P-A projection, the right cardiac margin is made up of the right atrium. As the right atrial margin is followed superiorly, a small notch is encountered. Superior to that, the image on the film is produced by the right lateral edge of the ascending aorta. Inferior to the right atrium is a curvilinear line that comprises the right lateral margin of the inferior vena cava. The left cardiac margin is composed of the left ventricle inferiorly, reaching to the level of the diaphragmatic leaf. As one follows the margin superiorly, he encounters the auricular appendage of the left atrium. Superior to this and lying above the left mainstem bronchus is the main pulmonary artery, which shows a small notch superiorly; above this lies the aortic arch (see Figs. 1-20 to 1-22). It is vital that the viewer remember the relationship of the chambers when he is using the oblique projections. These projections are of definite value in determining the status of the size of the individual chambers.

Right ventricular enlargement. An enlarged right ventricle impinges upon the sternum, producing rotation of the heart that is counterclockwise as viewed from

Text continued on p. 39.

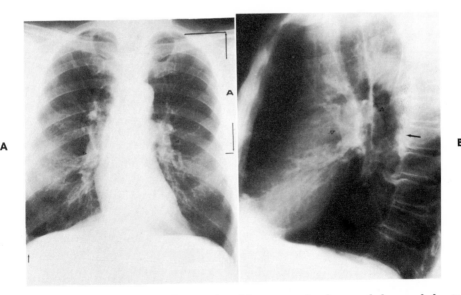

Fig. 1-27. Pulmonary disease may be manifested by increased volume and decreased density (emphysema). **A,** The left upper lobe (brackets, A) is observed to be more radiolucent than the right upper lobe with fewer vessels. There is some accentuated serration of the diaphragmatic leaf (lower arrow) as the result of the overexpansion of the lung. **B,** The lateral projection shows the large A-P diameter of the chest. The hilar vessels (open arrows) are quite prominent. This is an accompanying feature of emphysema. The solid arrow indicates advanced degenerative change of the thoracic spine as a result of aging. The heart appears round but small.

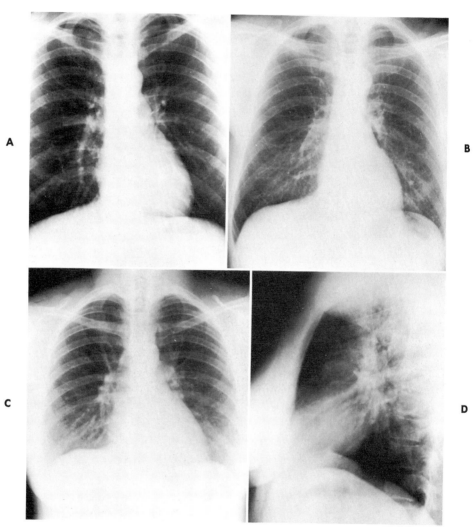

Fig. 1-28. A, Normal P-A chest, 23-year-old. **B,** Calcific focus in left lower lobe, with no acute disease or major abnormalities, 48-year-old male. **C,** P-A and **D,** lateral projections of a 35-year-old obese female. Broadening of the heart results from a high level of diaphragmatic leaves from the patient's habitus.

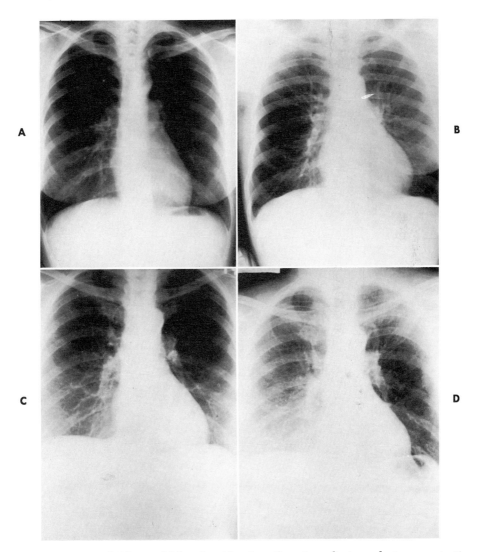

Fig. 1-29. A, Normal 34-year-old female with minor thoracic scoliosis producing accentuation of heart margins. **B,** Normal heart and lungs. The increased radiolucency of the right lower lobe is the result of removal of the right breast. **C,** Normal 70-year-old female with calcification of the aorta. **D,** Same patient following removal of the left breast; there is accentuated lucency of the left lung or increased density of the right lung.

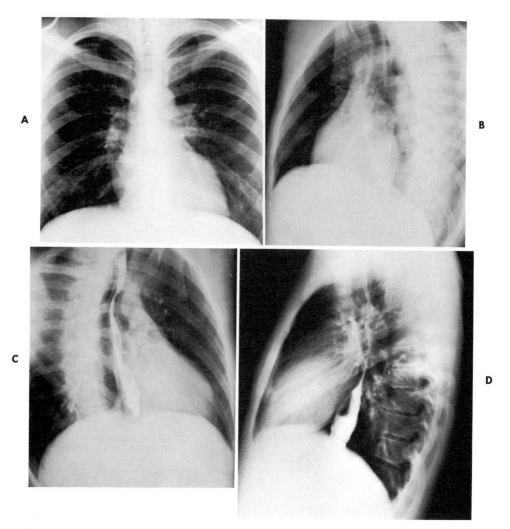

Fig. 1-30. Normal cardiac series in individuals of different habitus, with one appearing broad and the other small. These are normal variations of the appearance on the chest films.

E

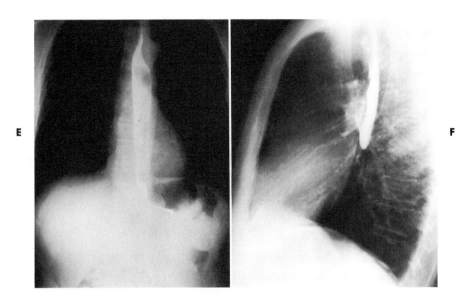

F

Fig. 1-30, cont'd. For legend see opposite page.

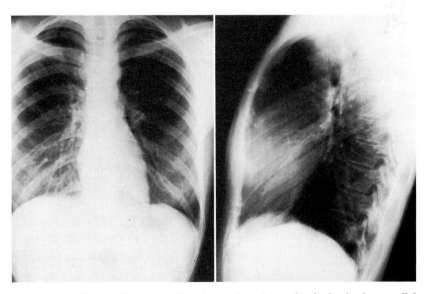

Fig. 1-31. Normal 27-year-old female. This is a rather thin individual who has small breasts that produce the ill-defined densities over the lower lobes.

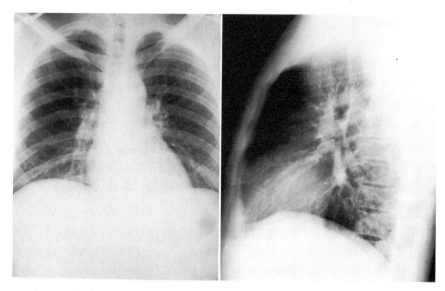

Fig. 1-32. Normal robust 30-year-old male.

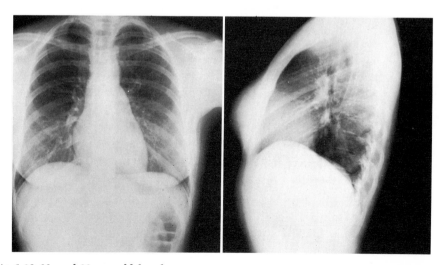

Fig. 1-33. Normal 23-year-old female.

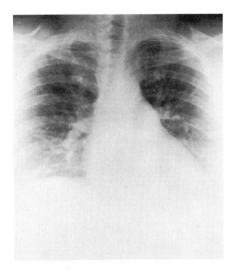

Fig. 1-34. Obese 32-year-old female.

above. An increased soft tissue density is produced in the radiolucent area (called the restrosternal clear space) just above the heart and behind the sternum. Other cardiovascular structures may also cause some increased density in this area, such as the right auricular appendage, an enlarged pulmonary artery, or even a very dilated aorta. The right anterior oblique projection gives a tangential view of this region. The notch at the base of the main pulmonary artery indicates the location of the pulmonary valves. (Fig. 1-35).

Left atrial enlargement. Anatomically, the left atrium is the most posterior superiorly placed chamber. It is in apposition to the esophagus and is the most easily assessed chamber. As it enlarges, the left atrium encroaches on the retro-cardiac space. This causes posterior and eventual right lateral displacement of the esophagus. The aorta prevents the esophagus from deviating to the left. The left mainstem bronchus is elevated by an enlarged left atrium. The right mainstem bronchus may be displaced to the right by a very large left atrium. As a result, the adjoining lung is compressed. Pulmonary disease caused by stasis may be the result of such compression. The left atrium is located posteriorly and pri-marily in the midline and left side. However, it must reach the right side of the chest in order to receive the right pulmonary veins. This, then, accounts for the changes in the right lung (Fig. 1-36).

Right atrial enlargement. In contrast to the left atrium, enlargement of the right atrium is more difficult to assess. Although the right atrium is the most right-sided chamber and potentially enlarges mostly to the right, any cardiac promi-nence to the right must be carefully studied. Scoliosis of the spine, rotation of the patient, high diaphragmatic level as a result of poor inspiratory effort, or intra-abdominal masses may cause the heart to be deviated and may produce an apparent enlargement of the right atrium. This point is illustrated well in the

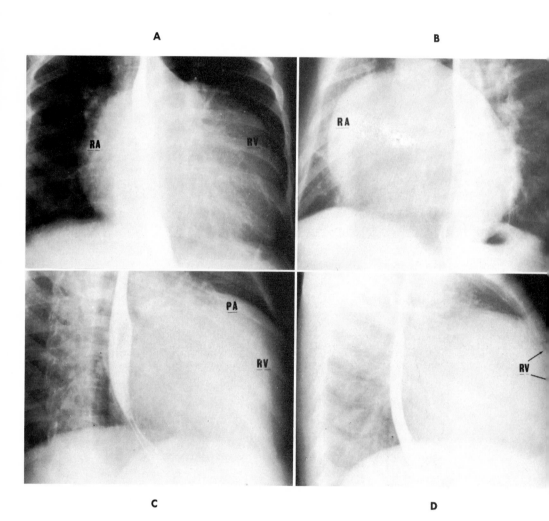

Fig. 1-35. Enlargement of the right ventricle may be marked. This individual has stenosis of the pulmonary valves and insufficiency of the tricuspid valve. **A,** P-A projection: the right atrium (*RA*) projects to the right of midline, but the right ventricle (*RV*) occupies the major portion of the left cardiac border. **B,** Left anterior oblique projection: the right atrium (*RA*) is quite rounded and projects along the superior margin of the right side of the heart. **C,** Left anterior oblique projection: the right ventricle (*RV*) and the pulmonary artery (*PA*) are observed to rise high along the left cardiac border. **D,** Lateral projection: the right atrium and the right ventricle (*RV*) occupy the retrosternal space and force the air-containing lung out of this region.

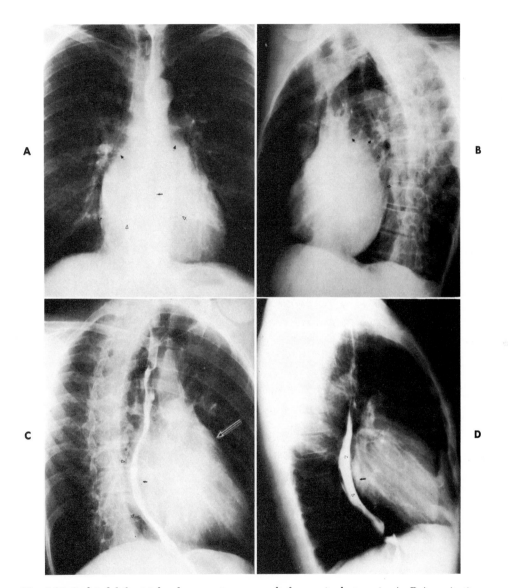

Fig. 1-36. Isolated left atrial enlargement may result from mitral stenosis. **A,** P-A projection: the left atrium is elevating the left and right mainstem bronchi (short solid arrow), deviating the barium filled esophagus to the right (long solid arrow) and projecting as a double shadow through the cardiac margin (open arrows). **B,** Left anterior oblique projection: the upper posterior margin of the heart is prominent (open arrows), indicating the area of the left atrium as it lies in apposition to the left mainstem bronchus (solid arrows) which is elevated. **C,** Right anterior oblique projection: the barium filled esophagus is displaced posteriorly and to the right (solid arrow) with the left atrium being sufficiently large to project beyond the esophagus (open arrows). The main pulmonary artery is large (outlined arrow). **D,** Lateral projection: the enlargement of the left atrium (solid arrow) encroaches on the anterior aspect of the barium filled esophagus (open arrows).

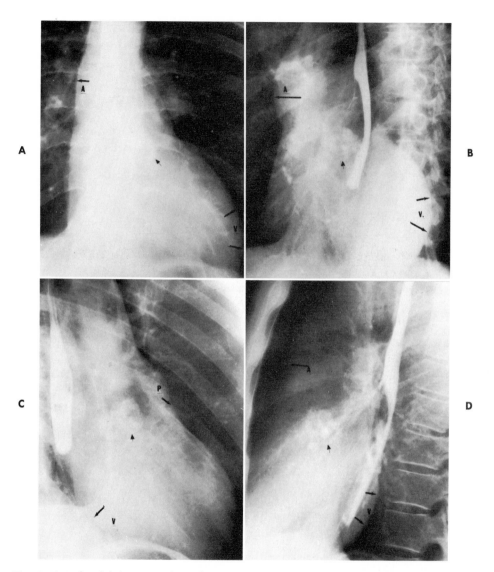

Fig. 1-37. Isolated left ventricular enlargement results, in this instance, from calcific aortic stenosis. **A,** In the P-A projection the ascending aorta is prominent, projecting to the right (*A*). Calcification in the aortic valve is observed (solid arrow). The left ventricular wall projects to the left (*V*). **B,** In the left anterior oblique projection the left ventricle (*V*) projects both backward and downward. The ascending aorta (*A*) is prominent, bulging anteriorly, superior to the calcified aortic valve (solid arrows). The direction of enlargement of the left ventricle indicates hypertrophy as well as dilation. **C,** On the right anterior oblique projection the left ventricle fills the infracardiac clear space (*V*-solid arrow). The calcific aortic valves are observed (solid arrow) and the main pulmonary artery (*P*) is prominent because of poststenotic dilatation of the aorta, which elevates the pulmonary artery. **D,** The lateral projection shows that the enlarged left ventricle projects behind the barium filled esophagus (*V*). The dilated aorta (*A*) and the calcific aortic valvulitis (solid arrows) are seen again.

expiration-inspiration P-A views. In the left anterior oblique projection, the right atrium is shown tangentially and comprises the right side of the cardiac outline. With right atrial enlargement, there is an increase in the soft tissue prominence in the right anterior superior portion of the cardiac outline.

Although it may appear simple to identify individual chamber enlargements, distortion in contour by enlargement of one chamber may produce sufficient cardiac distortion to simulate enlargement of a second chamber (Fig. 1-37).

Density. The roentgenographic density of the heart and blood vessels is normally soft tissue density, since the walls and the blood within absorb the same amount of x-rays. The most frequent cause for change in density is calcification. This is usually in the great vessels (Fig. 1-38) but may also occur in the heart and in the pericardium (Fig. 1-39). While it would seem that there would be an increased density with pericardial effusion, this is true only in comparison to the fat around the heart. There is a large amount of fat in the epipericardial areas normally. With pericardial effusion, the main changes are in size and configuration of the heart, but there are no changes in density. The differentiation between the soft tissue mass of the heart and the fat surrounding the heart can be used in identifying pericardial effusions if motion studies, such as cineroentgenographs, are used.

Roentgenographic functional evaluation of the heart requires study during the time of motion. This can be accomplished either by fluoroscopy or by recording a fluoroscopic image on x-ray movie film or videotape. The movement of the

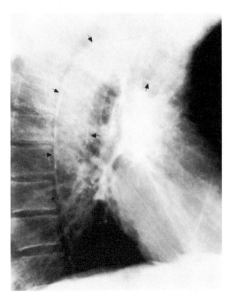

Fig. 1-38. Naturally occurring calcification produces a change in density. The aorta is extensively calcified (solid arrows). In addition, it is somewhat elongated, lying in apposition to the lung and making the margins apparent. This is the result of aging.

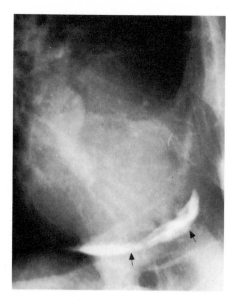

Fig. 1-39. Infection may induce calcification. There is extensive calcification along the pericardium overlying the base of the heart (solid arrows). When this occurs it is possible to define the exact margins of the pericardium.

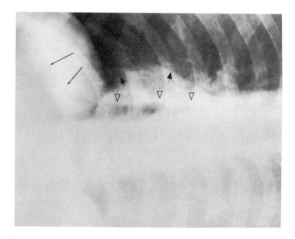

Fig. 1-40. Induced radiolucency may be utilized to evaluate the cardiac structures. Carbon dioxide has been introduced into the antecubital vein. Because the patient has been kept on the left side, the gas has collected in the right atrium (open arrows). The distance from the gas margin to the pericardiac outline (solid arrows) shows the amount of pericardial effusion. The gas has extended also into the hepatic veins (long solid arrows). (Courtesy of Dr. Walter Gaines, San Mateo, California)

heart is then studied for rhythm, rate, amplitude, and points of opposite pulsations which occur at the interspace between adjoining chambers, such as the left atrium and left ventricle.

Angiocardiography utilizes the artificially changed density of the heart with film recording of the appearance of the contrast medium to indicate specific abnormalities of the heart. The substances most frequently used for such studies are iodinated organic compounds; these are injected into the cardiac chambers or other great vessels by means of catheters placed in the veins or arteries. On occasion, the heart may also be studied by reducing the density. This is accomplished by injecting carbon dioxide into a vein of the arm; the carbon dioxide collects in the right atrium if the patient remains on his left side. This procedure shows the thickness of the wall and the overlying pericardium, enabling one to determine presence or absence of pericardial effusion or other pericardial or myocardial abnormalities (Fig. 1-40).

These various methods of studying the heart show distortions of anatomy reflected by the changes in size or contour. In study of the heart, the most frequently used projections are the P-A or A-P, a left lateral, and both right and left anterior oblique projections. The latter projections are specifically designed to allow a tangential view of the various surfaces of the heart. In this way it is possible to ascertain the disturbance of the contour of the heart and, thereby, evaluate a specific chamber abnormality. It is imperative that one know the location of the chambers in order to adequately use these views.

GREAT VESSELS

The great vessels include the superior and inferior vena cavae, the aorta with its major branches of the innominate artery, the carotid artery, the vertebral artery, the subclavian artery, the undivided segment of the main pulmonary artery, and the right and left main pulmonary arteries (Fig. 1-41). These vascular structures, together with the azygos vein, make up the vascular portion of the mediastinum, exclusive of the heart. The interrelationship of the positions to each other must be remembered if these structures are to be studied effectively. The pulmonary artery normally crosses in front of the base of the aorta, crossing from the right ventricle to the suprabronchial area above the left mainstem bronchus on the left, and then coursing somewhat to the right prior to its division into right and left main pulmonary arteries. The aorta, arising deep in the mass of the heart from the left ventricle, passes beneath the pulmonary artery and has superimposed upon it the right auricular appendage. The aorta courses superiorly and somewhat to the right to eventually swing back, in its horizontal or transverse portion, toward the left, crossing in front of the trachea, and turning inferiorly to lie along the left side of the mediastinum and esophagus. The superior vena cava descends along the right side of the mediastinum in close apposition to the ascending aorta, but it terminates in the right atrium somewhat superior to the point of exit of the aorta from the cardiac mass. The inferior vena cava is easily identified as it leaves the diaphragmatic surface, returning to the right atrium (Fig. 1-42). The inferior vena cava forms a crescent-shaped shadow which lies

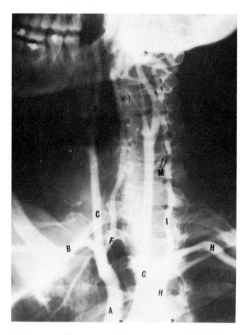

Fig. 1-41. Opacification of the vascular tree of the upper mediastinum, cervical area, and skull permits study of these anatomic structures. The major arterial trunks in the cervical area are demonstrated, with the innominate artery (*A*) dividing into the right subclavian artery (*B*), the right common carotid (*C*), and the right vertebral artery (*F*). The right internal carotid artery (*E*) and external carotid artery (*D*) rise out of the right common carotid (*C*). The left common carotid originates as a separate structure (*G*), bifurcating in its upper portion into the internal and external carotid with internal carotid passing through the petrous tip (top, small solid arrow). The left subclavian artery (*H*) originates separately, then continues in the sub-clavian area, giving off the left vertebral artery (*I*). As the vertebral artery passes through the foramina transversaria it may be narrowed by degenerative change about the spin (*M*, double arrows). The vertebral artery can be seen to pass through the foramen magnum and enter the skull. The width of the transverse foramina is shown by parallel lines along the margins of the vertebral artery. The right vertebral artery (*F*) passes through the transverse processes, lying lateral to the pedicle (set off by curved lines on the right side of the spine). All of these findings are normal.

at the cardiophrenic angle on the right as seen in the P-A projection, and overlies the inferior posterior aspect of the cardiac outline as seen in the lateral projection. Once identified, it can be located on most projections of the chest.

The size and configuration of the great vessels reflect both internal pressure and the tolerance of the vessel walls to this pressure. In other words, if peripheral obstruction with increased pressure exists, there will be a dilatation of the more proximal portion of the vessels. If, on the other hand, there is a proximal obstruction, such as valvular stenosis or shunting from the greater to the lesser circuit, there may well be a decreased diameter of the great vessels.

Aorta. The aorta's course has been described and can be identified on the routine films, particularly if the esophagus is filled with barium. The impression of the aortic arch on the trachea and the esophagus enables one to identify the

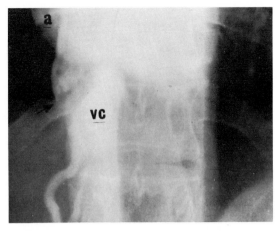

Fig. 1-42. The inferior vena cava (*VC*), as it enters the chest, produces a margin against the right lung and is used as a landmark in identifying the dimensions of the heart. The inferior vena cava has been opacified and the right atrium (*a*) is filling. The point of junction with the diaphragmatic leaf is indicated by the solid arrow.

right lateral aspect of the aortic arch. Aerated lung in contact with the left lateral aspect of the aortic arch demonstrates this margin. Dilatation of the aorta and of the brachiocephalic vessels indicates wall weakness or prolonged increased pressure. Systemic hypertension, for instance, produces primarily dilatation of the aorta. Coarctation would be one other cause of dilatation of the ascending aorta and of a portion of the descending aorta in the poststenotic areas. Poststenotic dilatation is a common finding in aortic valvular stenosis and apparently relates to the jet phenomenon, in which whirlpools are set up within the stream of blood, causing wall weakening and dilatation. Interruption of the force of the stroke volume of the ventricle, may, however, cause the more distal portions of the great vessels to remain smaller in diameter. In this instance, the aorta may appear hypoplastic. However, the hemodynamics of the circulation are such, that if there is an insufficiency of the aortic valve, the to and fro pulsation of the column of blood within the aorta will cause dilatation of the aorta.

Pulmonary arteries. Since the pulmonary arteries are surrounded by lung, they are visible to a great extent. Changes in the volume of these structures as well as of the pulmonary veins are, therefore, easily assessed roentgenographically. Thus, in pulmonary congestion, there may be dilatation of the vessels in both arterial and venous phases, owing to stasis. While a similar phenomenon may occur in the peripheral arteries of the systemic circulation, the changes are less evident since the vessels are surrounded by tissue of a similar density. Quantitative evaluation of decreased pulmonary venous size, however, becomes somewhat difficult. Decrease in size in the main pulmonary arterial segment indicates interruption of stroke volume to this vessel. This interruption usually comes from an obstruction of the outflow tract of the right ventricle, either at the valvular or infra-

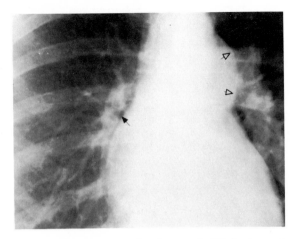

Fig. 1-43. The pulmonary vascularity may be decreased. While the main pulmonary artery (open arrows) is very large, the right main pulmonary artery (solid arrow) and the peripheral vessels are quite small. This results from pulmonary valvular stenosis with poststenotic dilatation. While the number of pulmonary vessels is the same, the small diameter indicates a decreased force of blood flow.

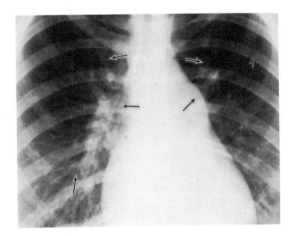

Fig. 1-44. The pulmonary vascularity is also a gauge to the cardiac status. The pulmonary arteries (open arrows) and pulmonary veins (solid arrows) are quite prominent. The aortic arch is small. This is indicative of increased flow through the pulmonary circuit and represents an abnormal communication between the left and right atrium.

valvular areas, or is caused by a failure of development of the artery, as in pulmonary atresia. (Fig. 1-43). Intracardiac obstructions at the level of the tricuspid valve may have a similar effect, since effective stroke volume of the right ventricle is reduced. If, on the other hand, excess blood is being carried by the pulmonary circulation from a left-to-right shunting within the heart, the pulmonary veins as well as the arteries may be dilated (Fig. 1-44).

Superior and inferior vena cavae. The superior and inferior vena cavae are either distorted by extrinsic pressure or dilated by intrinsic pressure. The actual size of the inferior vena cava is somewhat difficult to determine, since it is in close apposition to the heart and the diaphragmatic leaf and runs a very short course within the thoracic cavity. The superior vena cava, however, has a relatively long distance of travel within the thoracic cage; therefore, its margins and, to a certain extent, its size can be detected. Prevention of the return of blood to the right atrium from the systemic circulation will cause distention of the superior vena cava. This may be caused by extrinsic pressure, such as a tumor, either investing or compressing the superior vena cava or increased intracardiac pressure in the right atrium. This finding may, for instance, result from cardiac decompensation or heart failure. Excess blood may also reach the superior or inferior vena cava as a result of anomalous pulmonary veins returning to the right side of the circulation rather than to the left. This would then increase the volume present within the caval system, thereby causing some dilatation. Conversely, if there is obstruction to venous return at the diaphragmatic leaf, the inferior or superior vena cavae may be less apparent.

Respiratory system

Roentgenographic evaluation of the chest is most frequently used to demonstrate abnormalities in the lungs, since disease processes that cannot be detected by other physical examination methods can be seen on the roentgenogram. For example, the tumor nodule is well shown on the x-ray film in Fig. 1-45. This tumor nodule could not be discovered by any other method of routine physical examination. Oftentimes, the fact that the lungs represent only part of the total respiratory system is ignored. One should, therefore, in a systematic review of the chest film, identify the various components of this system: the lungs, the pleura, the hilar structures, the trachea, the mainstem bronchi, and the minor bronchi. The vascular components of the lungs have already been discussed; however, their presence and their configuration may also be of great assistance in interpreting the status of the lungs.

There is a usual segmentation pattern of the lungs which is outlined as follows:

I. Right lung
    A. Upper lobe (subsegments: apical, posterior, anterior)
    B. Middle lobe (subsegments: lateral, medial)
    C. Lower lobe (subsegments: superior, posterior basal, lateral basal, anterior basal and medial basal)

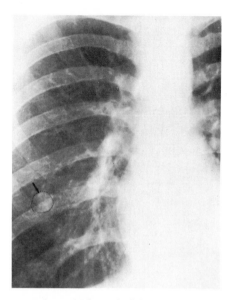

Fig. 1-45. A nodular density in the right lung (solid arrow). Such lesions are called "coin lesions." Their configuration and relative density, the appearance of surrounding lung tissue, and the number of such lesions are all parameters used to determine whether the densities represent old infection or neoplasm. In this instance, the density represents scarring from previous infection.

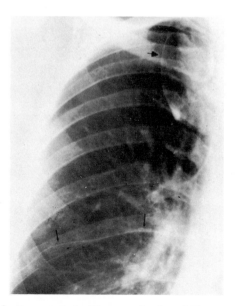

Fig. 1-46. An azygos lobe is present (solid arrows), shaped like a comma and representing a pleural reflection at the level of the azygos vein. The pleura is thickened along the horizontal fissure (lower small arrows), which defines the margin between the right upper and the right middle lobe. Fissures such as this are frequently radiodense in an older individual without indicating acute disease.

II. Left lung
   A. Upper lobe
      1. Subsegments: apical—posterior, anterior
      2. Lingula (subsegments: superior, inferior)
   B. Lower lobe (subsegments: superior, posterior basal, lateral basal, anterior medial basal)

Normally, there are ten subsegments of the right lung and eight subsegments of the left lung. Variation in segmentation is quite common and gives rise to accessory lobes. These accessory lobes represent portions of the other subsegments that are set off by pleural reflections. Some of the more common examples of this are azygos lobe, inferior medial basal segment, and segmental setoff of lingula as a separate lobe (Fig. 1-46). The azygos lobe stands as an excellent example of the effect of the vascular system on the respiratory system in something as gross as segmentation. The accessory azygos lobe results from a lateral position of the azygos vein, causing infolding of the pleural reflections into the lung.

Changes suggesting abnormalities

Detection of abnormalities in the lung by roentgenographic methods relies upon distortion of the anatomy by the disease process. The effect of the disease process is manifested by changes in size and density.

Size. The volume of the lung can be changed by collapse of a portion of the lung. This may result from obstruction to the airway, such as foreign body aspiration, tumor, or inflammatory stenosis of the bronchi. The effect is that the amount of lung which occupies a specific area of the hemithorax is reduced. This then, produces the rearrangement of the intrathoracic structures in order to occupy the space left by the reduction in size of a specific lobe (Fig. 1-47). The most easily accomplished change is overexpansion of adjoining lobes to occupy this space. One may, therefore, get compensatory emphysema. Mediastinal shift also occurs, as does some elevation of the diaphragmatic leaf.

Contraction of a lobe may occur from either intrinsic or extrinsic causes. A disease process that produces scarring and fibrosis within a lobe may, as in a patient with silicosis, produce progressive loss of volume as scar tissue develops. Changes in the pleura with contraction can also cause a relative loss of volume of a lobe. The volume of a portion of the lung may also be reduced by compression. Compression can, therefore, be considered as an extrinsic or extrapulmonary cause of loss of volume. The most frequent cause for decreased volume is poor inspiratory effort with resultant poor expansion of the lower lobe. Masses, either intrathoracic or subdiaphragmatic, pleural effusions, and deformities of the bony thorax (Fig. 1-48) all produce similar effects on the lungs. It should be remembered that the phenomenon of loss of volume is considered atelectasis. This is in contrast to the consolidation of pneumonia, in which some atelectasis may exist, but the major alteration is replacement of air by abnormal tissue and fluid; in atelectasis, air is prevented from reaching the alveoli and distal bronchi or is pushed out of them by extrinsic pressure.

Occasionally, the lung may be increased in size. Again, the most frequent

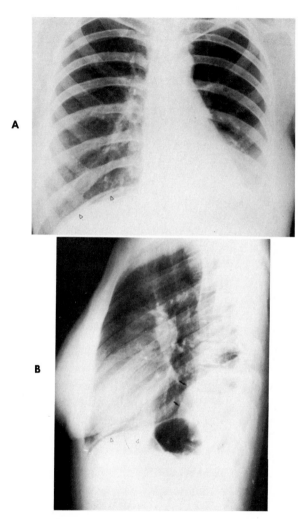

Fig. 1-47. A, The retrocardiac area is very white as seen in the P-A projection, and the medial aspect of the left hemidiaphragm cannot be seen. The left hilum is not identified; the ribs are closely approximated on the left. Beneath the right hemidiaphragm is a radiolucent crescent (open arrows). Atelectasis of the left lower lobe has occurred from a mucus plug in the bronchus. Previous surgery on the abdomen accounts for the free gas underneath the right hemidiaphragm (open arrows). **B,** On the lateral projection, the anterior margin of the atelectatic left lower lobe (solid arrows) is in contrast to the areated lung. The gas beneath the right hemidaphragm (open arrows) is again seen.

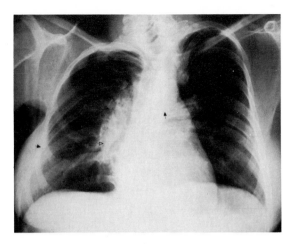

Fig. 1-48. Rather severe deformities of the skeletal structures may occur. In this instance, severe congenital scoliosis of the thoracic spine, convex to the right (open arrows), has reduced the total volume of the right lung. The ribs are bent (solid arrows) as the result of the prolonged scoliosis; the posterior ends of the left ribs lie in close apposition to each other. The left ribs, however, extend more laterally, allowing greater volume for expansion of the left side of the hemithorax. Individuals with this severe deformity may encounter cardiorespiratory difficulty.

cause for this increase is compensatory emphysema or overexpansion of a lung segment adjoining an atelectatic segment. This is nature's way of providing a balanced volume of tissue in each hemithorax. Other causes of overexpansion may relate to intrinsic diseases of the lungs, such as emphysema, emphysematous bullae, or obstructive emphysema. In this condition, air passes through the bronchi to the alveoli during inspiration, but because of some mechanism causing partial obstruction, the air cannot be forced out of the lung. Fluoroscopy in this condition will show a to-and-fro mediastinal swing. This results from the inability of one lung to collapse during expiration; the lung therefore remains as an enlarged soft tissue volume causing pressure against the mediastinum and depression of the diaphragmatic leaf on this side.

The change in size of a specific area of the lung may well produce alteration of the alignment of the internal structures of the lung. An example of this alteration is shown in Fig. 1-47, in which an atelectasis of the left lower lobe has produced a downward migration of the left hilar structures as well as a medial migration of the artery to the left lower lobe. A similar alteration in the orientation and position of the bronchi results from the change in the volume of a lobe. In addition, either the bronchi or arteries may be displaced by intrapulmonary disease.

Rather extensive work has been done on the location of the hilar structures, and it has been found that the left hilum normally lies at the level of, or slightly above, the right hilum. Change in the hilar level is a sensitive indicator of the loss of volume of lung segments. It should be remembered that the hila represent entrance to and, in part, drainage from the lung of the various structures and also indicate the site of pleural reflection from the visceral to the parietal pleura. The motion of the hila represents the ability of the lungs to function in terms of ingress and egress of air. There is a distinct pattern of motion of the hila during respiration. In expiration, the lower components of the hila tend to rotate upward and forward and at the same time are being displaced somewhat laterally by the pressure from the lower lobes. This is well illustrated in an expiration-inspiration P-A chest film (Fig. 1-23).

In addition to the changes in the level of the hila, alteration in the level of the normally occurring pleural reflections or fissures indicates change of volume. One rapidly becomes attuned to the usual level of the fissures, and deviation from their usual location becomes easily apparent. Although the description of the usual course of the fissures found in the standard anatomic textbooks is accurate, it is often difficult to apply to roentgenograms. Various projections and minor changes in the angle or plane of the course of the fissures alter the relation of the fissures to the adjoining osseous structures. Therefore, one relates the position of the fissures to the chest as a whole rather than to specific bony structures.

Density. A change in the usual radiolucency of the aerated lung is the most common indicator of abnormality. An increased density, as stated earlier, indicates the replacement of air by tissue, which absorbs radiation more effectively. As previously mentioned, however, there may be an excess amount of air present, thereby increasing the radiolucency of the lung. Increased density within the lung usually indicates excess soft tissue. This tissue may be tumor tissue, fibrosis, fluid, or blood. It is, therefore, necessary to use other criteria to determine, if possible, the true nature of this density. Some of the characteristics of the density which should be studied include number, size, configuration, uniformity of density, location within the lung, and, if possible, duration (Fig. 1-49). The configuration of the density, for instance, is wedge-shaped or tends to be slightly hemispherical with pulmonary infarction. Hemispherical densities located in the periphery of the lung with the flat surface of the hemisphere directed toward the pleura may well indicate an extrapulmonary or pleural origin of the density. A localized density which is spherical, indicating that all margins of the density can be seen, therefore, must be intrapulmonary. An atelectatic lobe is wedge-shaped, since the root of the lobe lies at the hilum and, as the peripheral portions of that lobe collapse, it tends to form a wedge pointing to the hilum. A smoothly lobulated or a lens-shaped density indicates that the consistency of the abnormal tissue is sufficiently soft to allow itself to be formed by the rather low pressure of the adjoining structures. Thus, encapsulated pleural effusion, cysts, or even intrapulmonary hemangiomas (Fig. 1-50) may form a configuration complying with the pressure of the adjoining structures.

The uniformity of the density of the abnormality is also important, and the most frequent alteration of uniformity is calcification. Calcific deposits within the central portion of a rounded radiodensity, for instance, would indicate that this is most likely the result of a previous infection (Fig. 1-51). Certain tumors, such as metastatic osteogenic sarcoma, or even some of the benign tumors, such as

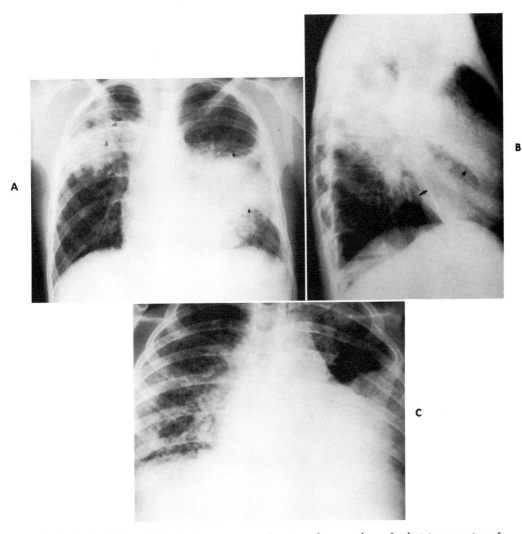

Fig. 1-49. **A,** Infiltrate into the lung removes the air and causes loss of adjoining margins of adjacent organs. There is pneumonia present in the lingular division of the left upper lobe (solid arrows) which has caused loss of the margin of the left side of the heart. The right upper lobe shows consolidation with air bronchograms (open arrows). This indicates loss of aeration of the alveoli, but with patent bronchi. **B,** The lateral projection shows the area of infiltrate to occupy the lingular division of the left upper lobe (short solid arrow). Some fluid is observed along the course of the oblique fissure (lower solid arrow). **C,** Diffuse pulmonary disease is seen, with a nodular pattern representing pulmonary edema, in this instance, the result of renal failure.

**Fig.
1-50**

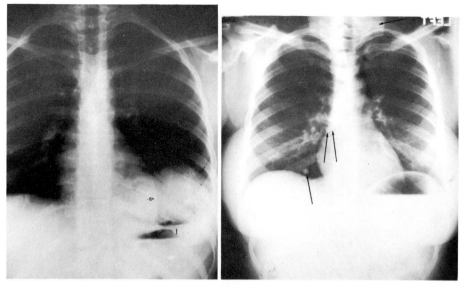

**Fig.
1-51**

Fig. 1-50. The overall appearance of the density within the lung assists in determining its nature. The margination of this mass is smooth, although somewhat lobulated. Its density is irregular, with the lower portion of it being radiolucent. It has not obscured the heart margin (open arrows), indicating that it lies behind the heart. The gas bubble of the stomach lies in close apposition to the lung (solid arrow), indicating that there is no major pleural effusion. When the P-A projection is used in conjunction with lateral and other views, the consistency of the mass is shown to be relatively soft. This represents a hemangioma of the lung.

Fig. 1-51. A calcific focus is present in the lung, and calcified foci in the right hilum indicate old inflammatory disease. A cervical rib is present on the left (long solid arrow).

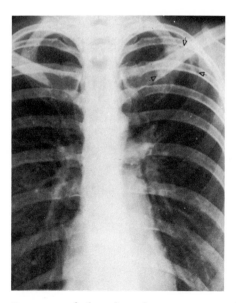

Fig. 1-52. Change in density may result from loss of aeration surrounding increased aeration. There is a cavity in the left apex (open arrows) as the result of acute infection by coccidioidomycosis, a fugus disease endemic in several areas of the west and southwest.

A   B

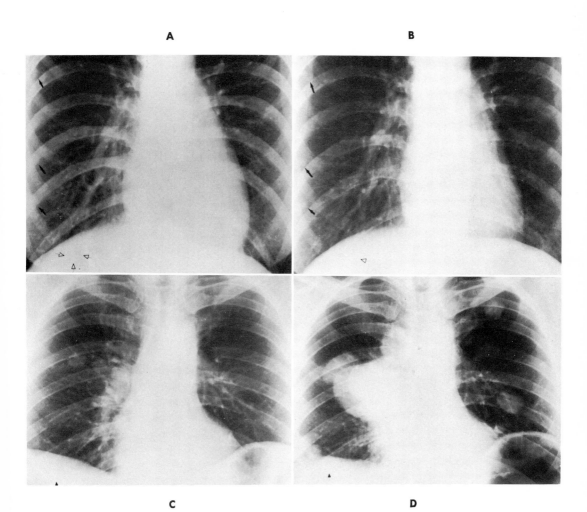

C   D

Fig. 1-53. A, The P-A projection of the chest in 1962 shows multiple nodular lesions in the lung (solid arrows). Hidden behind the right hemidiaphragm is a large lesion (open arrows). **B,** In 1966 the nodular densities (solid arrows) are appreciably smaller and the retrodiaphragmatic lesion (open arrow) much smaller. This represents successful treatment of metastatic carcinoma of the thyroid. The multiplicity of the lesions and the clinical history established the diagnosis. **C,** In contrast, the retrodiaphragmatic lesion on the right (solid arrow), in this case, has in two years expanded appreciably. **D,** There are now extensive masses present in both lungs and in the right hilar area. The right cardiac margin is no longer visible. This represents progression of metastatic disease but of a very slowly growing type.

hamartoma, may contain calcific deposits as well, but the deposits are not usually as focal and discreate as those resulting from a previous infection. Cavitation within the central portion of a density is manifested by increased radiolucency (Fig. 1-52). This indicates communication with the bronchus, since a cavity that does not communicate with the bronchus is filled with fluid and cannot be distinguished from a solid mass of other tissue. The status of the lung adjoining the focal density—evidence of infiltration into the tissue, adjoining scarring, and overlying pleural thickening—would be supportive evidence of an inflammatory lesion. Displacement of adjacent structures would indicate a growing mass such as a tumor.

A single nodular density without findings or a previous history of other systemic disease, particularly neoplasm, will most frequently be inflammatory in origin. If there are multiple nodular densities throughout the lung, the most common etiology will be metastatic tumor. The duration of the abnormality is detectable only by comparison with serial films. The duration of a lesion is perhaps the most vital finding in determining the nature of the process and whether the disease is stable (Fig. 1-53).

It is possible to alter the normal radiodensities of the lung and the pleura by artificially changing such densities. Contrast medium may be instilled into the trachea and thence into the bronchi and alveoli to define the internal structure of the bronchi and trachea. The patency of the bronchi may, of course, also be determined by this procedure. The size of the bronchi may be increased or de-

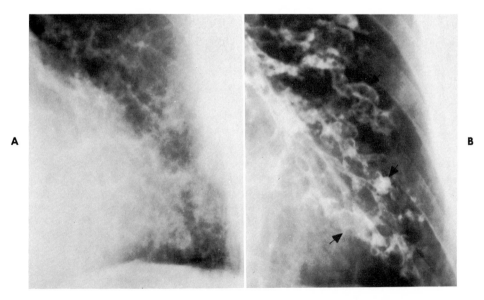

Fig. 1-54. A, Detailed films of the lingular division of the left upper lobe show irregular linear and curvilinear densities within the lungs. **B,** Instillation of iodinated compound into the bronchi (bronchogram) shows the irregular densities to be thickened walls of bronchi. The bronchi (solid arrows) and alveoli are dilated in this area, indicative of bronchiectasis.

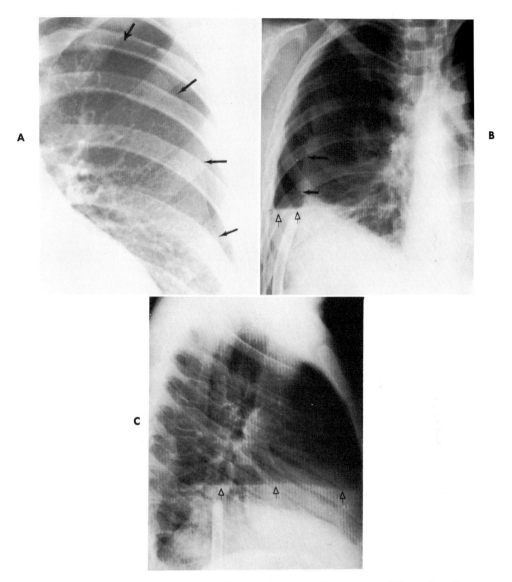

Fig. 1-55. A, The outer margin of the lung (solid arrows) is separated from the rib cage. The radiolucency of the space between the lung and the ribs indicates air, in this instance, a spontaneous pneumothorax. The pleura appears as a solid, fine, white line (tip of the arrows), when it is in apposition to air on both sides. **B,** If fluid and air are both present in the pleural space, an air-fluid level (open arrows) is seen. In the P-A projection the margin of the partly collapsed lung contrasting against the air in the pleural space is observed (solid arrows). A radiopaque drainage tube extends into the pleural space to attempt to remove the fluid and the air. **C,** The lateral projection shows the extent of the air-fluid level in its anteroposterior axis (open arrows).

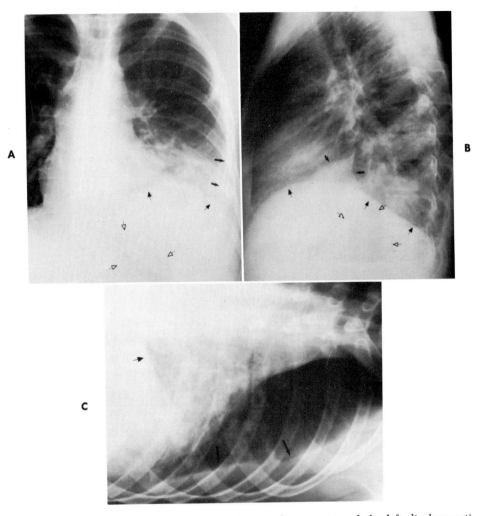

Fig. 1-56. A, In the erect P-A projection the left cardiac margin and the left diaphragmatic leaf are not identifiable and there is increased density in the left lower hemithorax. This represents fluid collection within the pleural space, with what appears to be the diaphragmatic leaf (solid, short-tailed arrows) being separated appreciably from the gas bubble of the stomach (open arrows). Increased density is present laterally (broad solid arrows). **B,** On the lateral projection the broad solid arrows indicate the extension of fluid into the oblique fissure. The gas bubble of the stomach (open arrows) is seen to be appreciably below the aerated lung. **C,** Placing the patient on his side shows that the fluid (long solid arrows) extends cephalad, separating the lung from the ribs and showing the amount of fluid. The true level of the left hemidiaphragm (short solid arrows) is now seen. The use of gravity enables determination of the amount of fluid.

creased. The former is considered bronchiectasis (Fig. 1-54), the latter, bronchial stenosis by compression, tumor, or postinflammatory scarring. Diagnostic pneumothoraces may also be used to determine the configuration of the pleural space and the outer margins of the lungs (Fig. 1-55). If pleural effusion is present, an excess amount of radiodensity is present in the area of the pleural space. This may obscure the heart, it increases the distance of the aerated lung from the gas bubble of the stomach, and it reduces the sharp angularity of the costophrenic sulci. Because of gravity, there is a shift in the density concomitant with the change in the body position. Therefore, pleural effusion, which initially is hidden in the lower portion of the chest, may be brought into better view in the upper portion of the chest by placing the patient on his side and obtaining another film (Fig. 1-56).

One is accustomed to seeing the margins of the heart and of the diaphragmatic leaves because the aerated lung is in apposition to these structures. If such aeration is lost, the margin of the adjoining structure is obscured. This is called the silhouette sign and is extremely useful in detecting disease in a small volume of the lung.

Mediastinum and digestive system

The digestive system is not ordinarily one of the systems considered in viewing the plain chest film. It must be remembered, however, that the gas bubble of the stomach is usually easily identifiable on both P-A and lateral projections of the chest. The splenic flexure of the colon is often outlined by gas. The esophagus, of course, is one of the prime structures of the chest, and when the esophagus is opacified with barium, it is used to evaluate the status of the mediastinal structures. Intrinsic lesions of the esophagus also produce abnormalities on the plain chest film. The course of the esophagus is usually studied by means of the ingestion of barium; however, a catheter may be placed in the esophagus to show its course, and occasionally the esophagus can be identified when filled with air.

In individuals with achalasia, the esophagus may be grossly dilated and project to the right of the mediastinum as a soft tissue mass as seen in the plain films (Fig. 1-57). An air-fluid level in the posterosuperior mediastinal area also results from achalasia with distention. Hiatus hernia is a fairly frequent abnormality identifiable on a plain film of the chest (Fig. 1-58). The hiatus hernia presents as a rounded soft tissue density with an air-fluid level lying at the retrocardiac space and projecting through the heart shadow.

If the esophagus is to be studied adequately, it is obviously necessary to change its density artificially. The esophagus cannot be thoroughly studied unless there is an evaluation of its function as well as its form. Fluoroscopic evaluation can be recorded by means of cineroentgenography or videotape recording. This enables one to restudy, at leisure and at varying speeds, an event as it occurs.

Seldom does the esophagus remain opacified in its entirety, with or without distention, unless there is either obstruction to the passage of barium or decreased

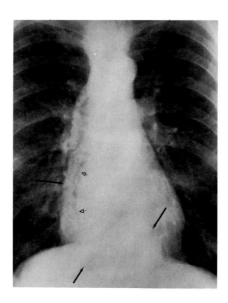

Fig. 1-57. On a routine chest film, the mediastinum appears irregular, projecting toward the right (upper long arrow). This represents a markedly dilated esophagus as the result of narrowing at the junction of the esophagus and the stomach (achalasia). The actual cardiac margin (open arrows) overlies the esophagus. In addition, a rounded density (lower long arrows) lies within the retrocardiac area. This represents a very dilated and tortuous aorta. The contrasted soft tissue density against the air-filled lung enables the diagnosis to be made.

motility of the esophagus. The demonstration of a consistently outlined esophagus on several films in a series, with or without distention, should raise suspicion of impaired functional ability (Fig. 1-59). Such a finding may be an incidental observation on a chest film which, for example, has been obtained for the evaluation of heart size. This finding would indicate the necessity for more definitive esophageal studies. Stenosis, achalasia, and carcinoma can all produce obstruction and dilatation. Scleroderma, inanition, and myasthenia gravis are three conditions that can produce loss of motility of the esophagus.

Besides being dilated, the esophagus may be distorted by either intrinsic or extrinsic processes. For example, cardiac enlargement, particularly in the region of the left atrium, will initially displace the esophagus posteriorly and then to the right. This displacement may cause some general narrowing of the esophagus over the cardiac margin. Most of the adjoining disease processes produce a deformity, either by adhesions, as with traction diverticulum at the level of the hilum, or by focal pressure such as that caused by subcarinal lymph node enlargement. Deformity of the esophagus by the aorta is very common. The tortuous aorta crosses from the left side of the hemithorax to lie in the prevertebral area and passes through an opening in the diaphragmatic leaf to enter the abdomen. The resulting esophageal deformity lies on the posterior wall of the esophagus, in contrast to the deformity produced by the cardiac outline. Normally, the aortic arch produces some deformity along the left lateral wall of the

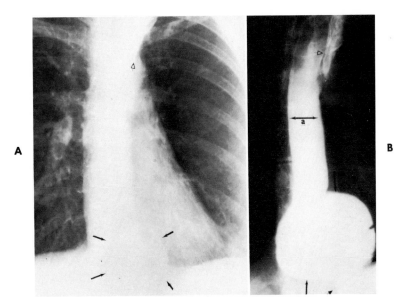

Fig. 1-58. A, A rounded density is seen in the retrocardiac area (solid arrows). In the upper portion of this mass is a small radiolucency. **B,** When barium is placed in the esophagus it is observed to widen (double-ended arrow, *a*) and the large sac fills in the lower end of the esophagus (broad, solid arrow). This represents a herniation of the fundus of the stomach into the thoracic cage (hiatus hernia) through the esophageal hiatus (short solid arrow). It is identified on the P-A projection (**A**) when it is in contact with the aerated lung. The density of the upper mediastinum (open arrow) represents a densely calcified pleural plaque from old inflammatory disease.

esophagus. It is this deformity that enables one to adequately identify the medial aspect of the aortic arch. In addition, adjoining abnormalities may cause dilatation of the esophagus by producing obstruction. The esophagus may also be delayed in emptying as a result of obstruction. In instances of this type of displacement or deformity, definitive studies of the esophagus show that the mucosal pattern of the esophagus is intact and that there is a lack of interruption of the primary or secondary peristaltic waves. In contrast, the deformities resulting from intrinsic disease of the esophagus usually show irregularity of the lumen of the esophagus and, most frequently, distortion of the lining of the esophagus. Narrowing, obstruction, or interruption of normal peristalsis all may reflect intrinsic disease as well. The contour of the esophagus demonstrated on the roentgenograms may be grossly altered by intrinsic disease. Spasm, as in esophagitis, or tertiary contractions or corkscrew esophagus, resulting from myoneural dysfunction are two examples. Alteration of the contour of the esophagus by intrinsic disease is a condition frequently evident in the older individual and may or may not produce delay of the passage of barium through the distal esophagus. Distinction between these irregularities and varices of the esophagus can be made if one remembers that when the esophagus is distended, tertiary contractions disappear, whereas esophageal varices persist.

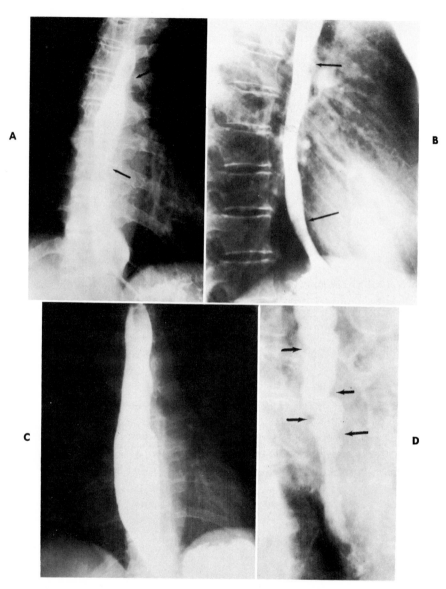

Fig. 1-59. The esophagus is most easily evaluated by opacifying it with barium sulfate suspension. **A,** The normal esophagus in the A-P projection shows impression on its lumen by the left mainstem bronchus (upper arrow) at the level of the posterior aspect of the heart (middle arrow) and at the cardioesophageal junction (lowest arrow). **B,** On the lateral projection the area of impression at the left mainstem bronchus and retrocardiac area (solid arrows) is again seen. These are normal physiologic narrowings. In addition, there is usually narrowing at the level of the aortic arch. **C,** If the esophagus is relatively immobile, as in scleroderma, the diameter is uniformly broad and peristaltic activity is very slight. A relatively smooth, constantly opacified esophagus showing only the expected narrowing from extrinsic pressure is indicative of loss of muscular action. **D,** By contrast, the esophagus in the older individual may undergo severe irregular contractions which are not propulsive. These are considered tertiary contractions and are irregular in form and location (arrows); they are not seen when the esophagus is distended.

Other mediastinal structures

Other organ systems are present in the mediastinum as well, and these include lymph nodes, the neurofibrous mesenchymal tissues, and the thymus. The most common abnormality of these structures that can be seen on the chest film is enlargement. One of the key findings to be observed is a silhouette sign as applied to the normal structures. Thus, the superior margin of the aortic arch may be obscured by superior mediastinal lymph node enlargement. The right or left cardiac margin may appear lobulated or seem to be absent as a result of anterior mediastinal masses such as thymus or lymph nodes (Fig. 1-60). The descending aortic margin, usually lying in apposition to the left lower lobe, may be obscured by paravertebral retropleural soft tissues, such as neurofibromas.

The location of the mass relative to the mediastinum is very important in interpreting the nature of the abnormality. The thymus and lymph nodes are located in the anterior mediastinal compartment, and teratoid tumors also occur there. Lipomas, angiomas, and perhaps cysts would be considered among the teratoid tumors. These, in the case of lipomas, are hyperlucent. Angiomas and teratomas may be partially calcified; such calcification represent phleboliths or bone elements. Lymph nodes, bronchogenic cysts, and duplication cysts of the

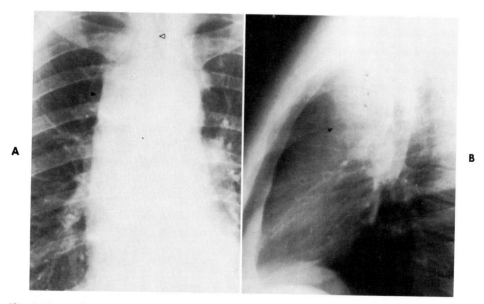

Fig. 1-60. A, Abnormalities of the lymphatic system are shown by increased soft tissue density in the region of the nodes. The mediastinum is diffusely broad, with the right side of the mediastinum (solid arrow) particularly affected. The trachea (open arrows) shows compression from the superior extension of the lymph nodes. The major portion of the aorta is obscured, as is the superior cardiac margin. **B,** In the lateral projection the anterior margin of the superior mediastinal mass (solid arrow) extends into the retrosternal clear space. Soft tissue enlargement in the retrosternal area along the course of the internal mammary lymph nodes represents diffuse involvement of the mediastinal lymphatics by Hodgkins' disease.

gastrointestinal tract will be found in the midportion of the mediastinum, in association with the bronchi. Posteriorly, primary disease processes of a tumorous nature would most likely be neurogenic or fibrous in origin. Again, inflammatory disease originating in the region of the spine or in the posterior mediastinum may simulate primary tumors.

Assessment of mediastinal abnormalities also implies evaluation of the contour of mediastinal contents. The density should be studied to determine whether it is smoothly marginated, lobulated, isolated, multiple, or calcified. If at all possible, the duration of the disease process should be determined. For example, by studying the nature of the density of the abnormality, it can be seen that the rather large azygos nodes and lobulated hilar nodes in sarcoid have a tendency to develop less matting of the lymph nodes than in the lymphomas (Fig. 1-61). The isolated and poorly defined hilar or mediastinal mass raises the possibility of metastatic tumor. One must continually be cautious, however, that the presence of the mass is not oversuggested when, in actuality, what is being identified is a prominent azygos vein, a prominent superior vena cava, or evidence of senescent changes of the vascular structures.

The contour of the trachea at the thoracic inlet as well as the form of the esophagus is of importance in evaluating the superior anterior mediastinum. This is the area most frequently involved by retromanubrial and retrosternal extension of thyroid enlargement.

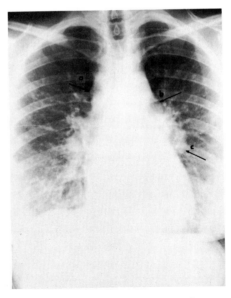

Fig. 1-61. Patterns of lymph node enlargement may be indicative of certain diseases. The azygos node (*a*) is enlarged, as is the left suprahilar node (*b*). These, together with the rounded enlarged infrahilar nodes and the peribronchial nodes (*c*), are the findings expected with Boeck's sarcoid. The peripheral pulmonary parenchyma also shows linear and nodular densities indicative of involvement of the lungs by sarcoid.

REQUIRED READINGS

Felson, B.: Fundamentals of chest roentgenology, Philadelphia, 1960, W. B. Saunders Company.

Squire, L. F.: Fundamentals of roentgenology, Cambridge, 1964, Harvard University Press.

RECOMMENDED READINGS

Caffey, J.: Pediatric x-ray diagnosis; section II, the thorax, Chicago, 1961, Year Book Medical Publishers, Inc.

Paul, L. W., and Juhl, J. H.: The essentials of roentgen interpretation; section V, the chest, New York, 1964, Hoeber Medical Division, Harper & Row, Publishers.

Schwedel, J. B.: Clinical roentgenology of the heart, New York, 1946, Paul B. Hoeber.

ADDITIONAL READINGS

Leigh, T. F., and Weens, H. S.: The mediastinum, Springfield, Illinois, 1959, Charles C Thomas, Publisher.

Templeton, F. E.: X-ray examination of the stomach, Chicago, 1944, University of Chicago Press.

2

ABDOMEN

Summary of basic concepts

Naturally occurring contrast in the abdomen is less than in the chest. Interrelationship between organ systems should be considered; for example, renal calculi and secondary hyperparathyrodism from malabsorption syndrome with osteomalacia. Signs of these various diseases may be evident on a single film of the abdomen. Major components are the musculoskeletal, gastrointestinal, hepatopancreatic, lymphatic system and spleen, and genitourinary systems.

I. Musculoskeletal system
  A. Components
    1. Lumbar spine
    2. Pelvis
    3. Hip joints and proximal femora
    4. Lower ribs
    5. Thoracolumbar spine
    6. Sacrum
    7. Coccyx
    8. Sacroiliac joints
  B. Parameters lumbar spine, pelvis, sacrum, proximal femora
    1. Density
      a. Naturally occurring—increased
        (1) Degenerative change
        (2) Metastasis
        (3) Metabolic disease
        (4) Developmental aberration
        (5) Paget's disease
      b. Naturally occurring—decreased
        (1) Inflammatory disease
        (2) Osteoporosis
        (3) Osteomalacia
        (4) Tumor primary or secondary
          (a) Bones most frequently involved by metastatic disease
          (b) Epidural plexus and vascularity of these structures cause frequent tumor deposit
      c. Density—artifically changed (myelography)—lumbar spine
        (1) Introduction of contrast medium into subarachnoid space
          (a) Increased by using iodinated medium
          (b) Reduced by using air
          (c) Contrasts against soft tissues around dura and bone of spine
        (2) Parameters
          (a) Filling of nerve root cuffs

    (b) Alignment of nerve roots

    (c) Smoothness of margin of contrast column

    (d) Mobility of column

    (e) Continuity of column

   (3) Extradural abnormalities within the spinal canal change contour of the contrast column

   (4) Abnormalities within dural tube interrupt column

2. Contour

  a. Change from aging (degeneration) of disc, vertebral body and pelvis

   (1) Most frequent site in spine

   (2) Spurs around margins

   (3) Narrow sacroiliac joints

  b. Change from inflammatory arthritis

   (1) Ankylosing spondylitis

   (2) Rheumatoid arthritis

   (3) Other inflammation

   (4) Change in contour and density—vertebrae, posterior joints of the spine, sacroiliac joints

  c. Change from trauma

   (1) Compression

   (2) Split (seat belt fractures—lumbar spine)

  d. Change from malalignment

   (1) Spine

    (a) Wedged on concavity (b) Posterior elements—adaptive form

   (2) Pelvis—adaptive shaping

3. Number—spinal segments

  a. Five lumbar segments—usual

  b. Fewer or more true lumbar segments—frequent

4. Alignment—lumbar spine

  a. Scoliosis (lateral curvature)

   (1) Spasm

   (2) Idiopathic

   (3) Congenital (hemivertebra)

   (4) Acquired (fracture, leg length discrepancy, etc.)

  b. Lordosis (anterior curvature)

   (1) Usual alignment

   (2) Related to posture

   (3) Decreased in spasm

   (4) True degree seen on lateral film in erect position

5. Evaluation of discs

  a. Size

   (1) Increases from first lumbar to fourth lumbar

   (2) Fifth lumbar may be smaller normally

  b. Contour: wedge shaped—narrow posteriorly

  c. Density

   (1) Normal

    (a) Soft tissue—usual

    (b) Calcification (increase) or gas (decreased) in degeneration

(2) Artificially increased (discograms)

    (a) Normal—contrast medium remains within disc

    (b) Ruptured—escape of medium outside disc margins

  6. Evaluation of small posterior joints of spine and transverse process

    a. Oblique projections most useful

    b. Form of joint facets clue to functional aspect of spine

    c. Abnormalities of transverse processes frequently missed because not carefully studied

C. Evaluation lower ribs and costocartilages

  1. Overlie upper abdomen

  2. Costocartilage calcifications resemble intra-abdominal calculi (think from skin to skin in evaluating roentgenographs)

  3. Postoperative changes of twelfth rib occasionally the only roentgenographic clue to renal surgery if renal outline simulated by residual renal bed after nephrectomy

D. Heavy musculature of lumbar spine and retroperitoneal space

  1. Psoas margins and abdominal musculature evident on films of abdomen

  2. Loss of definition of psoas margins: abnormality of retroperitoneal space

  3. Density

    a. Naturally occurring (radiolucent)—normal

      (1) Fat in retroperitoneal area contrasts against other soft tissue; invests muscular borders of abdomen

      (2) Loss of fat decreases margination of retroperitoneal structure

    b. Naturally occurring (radiolucent)—abnormal: free intraperitoneal air

      (1) Perforation of hollow viscus

      (2) Postoperative state

      (3) Air will rise to upper portion of abdomen

        (a) Free air beneath diaphragm (erect film)

        (b) Gas beneath anterior abdominal wall with patient lying on back

    c. Density—artificially reduced

      (1) Peritoneal cavity (pneumoperitoneum—enables evaluation of intra-abdominal structures)

      (2) Retroperitoneal (presacral air insufflation—shows kidneys and adrenal glands)

II. Hepatopancreatic system (interaction between these two structures frequent component of disease)

A. Liver (parameters)

  1. Size

    a. Enlarged

      (1) Most frequent abnormality

      (2) From infiltration, congestion or excess tissue (tumor)

      (3) Changes location of structures adjoining

      (4) Margin seen against adjoining fat

    b. Small

      (1) Cirrhosis

      (2) Right kidney elevated

  2. Density

      a. Normal—soft tissue
      b. Naturally occurring abnormal
         (1) Calcification within cysts, metastasis or calculi
         (2) Radiolucent (gas) from biliary fistula
      c. Artificially increased
         (1) Intravenous cholangiogram
            (a) Contrast medium excreted from liver through ductal system
            (b) Gallbladder seen from passive opacification
         (2) Transhepatic cholangiography
         (3) Oral Cholecystography
            (a) Evaluates ability of gallbladder to concentrate contrast medium
            (b) Reveals irregularity of size, failure of filling, displacement, irregular filling

  B. Pancreas (parameters)
    1. Size
      a. Delineated by adjoining structures: stomach, duodenum, colon
      b. Structures displaced or deformed if pancreas enlarged
    2. Density
      a. Abnormal density (calcifications)
         (1) Inflammation
         (2) Tumor
      b. Artificially increased
         (1) Vascular injection
         (2) Contrast medium forced into ducts

III. Gastrointestinal tract
  A. Artificially induced change in contrast
    1. Specific studies for specific structures
      a. Upper gastrointestinal series—stomach, duodenum, proximal jejunum
      b. Small bowel series—duodenum, jejunum, ileum
      c. Barium enema and pneumocolon—colon, distal ileum
    2. Internal structure of the viscus is the only part demonstrated
    3. External wall of viscus demonstrated by special technique
      a. Pneumoperitoneum
      b. High kilovoltage roentgenographic technique
  B. Parameters
    1. Form
      a. Smooth or irregular—tumor or ulcer
      b. Abnormal configuration of wall
         (1) Retraction—adhesion or scar
         (2) Protrusion—diverticula
    2. Consistency
      a. Pliable or rigid (infiltrated)
      b. Mobile or fixed (by adjoining abnormality)
    3. Function
      a. Peristalsis
         (1) Depth
         (2) Number of waves—hyperactive, hypoactive or normal
         (3) Symmetry of waves

    b. Utilize fluoroscopy, cineroentgenography, videotape recording, pressure recordings

    c. Disturbed by

      (1) Extrinsic disease

      (2) Intrinsic disease

4. Continuity

    a. Interrupted by obstruction or abnormal motility

    b. Abnormal communication

      (1) Fistula

      (2) Postoperative

5. Mucosal pattern (lining of viscus)

    a. Destruction

      (1) Ulcer

      (2) Tumor

    b. Infiltration

      (1) Thickened and irregular

      (2) Tumor

      (3) Inflammatory reaction

      (4) Edema

    c. Atrophy

    d. Excess

      (1) Polyp

      (2) Edema or tumor

    e. Demonstration of lining

      (1) Double contrast

        (a) Lining of viscus coated with barium

        (b) Viscus then distended with air

          (i) Positive contrast delineation of polyps surrounded by negative contrast of air

          (ii) With positive contrast alone, polyps appear as negative shadows

      (2) Less contrast material

        (a) Displaced by intentional compression of viscus to show lining

        (b) Evacuation film of barium enema for demonstration of mucosa of colon

6. Location

    a. Indicator of masses within abdomen

    b. Distortion of position: apparent, congenital, retracted, or displaced

7. Abnormal density

    a. Ingestion of opaque, nonmedicinal substance, such as foreign bodies or contrast medium as for gallbladder study

    b. Abnormal lucency of wall: pneumatosis cystoides intestinalis

    c. Calcification: meconium ileus peritonitis

    d. Extravasation of contrast medium from ruptured viscus

8. Initial examination with plain film

    a. Air-fluid levels demonstrate abnormality of motility

    b. Lining may be outlined by intraluminal gas

9. Order of study of upper gastrointestinal series

a. Esophagus
b. Cardioesophageal junction
c. Gastric fundus
d. Pars media
e. Antrum of stomach
f. Prepyloric region of stomach
g. Pyloric canal
h. Duodenal bulb
i. Descending limb of duodenum
j. Ampulla of Vater
k. Horizontal limb of duodenum
l. Ligament of Treitz
m. Proximal jejunum
n. If small bowel opacified: jejunum, ileum, and cecum in that order

10. Determinations from upper gastrointestinal series
    a. Function of intestinal tract reflected in change of contour
    b. Continuity of barium column in small bowel indicates motility of meal
    c. Distance between the filled lumen of adjoining loops of small bowel indicates thickness of wall
    d. Distance between stomach and transverse colon increased with perigastric masses
    e. Artifical density decreased with excess intraluminal fluid from:
       (1) Obstruction
       (2) Residual from enema
       (3) Ingestion of fluid just prior to examination

11. Order of study of colon (barium enema)
    a. Rectum
    b. Rectosigmoid
    c. Sigmoid
    d. Descending colon
    e. Splenic flexure
    f. Transverse colon
    g. Hepatic flexure
    h. Ascending colon
    i. Cecum
    j. Ileocecal valve
    k. Terminal ileum
    l. Appendix

12. Determinations from colon examination
    a. Normally angles and narrows at change of peritoneal relation: rectosigmoid, descending colon, splenic flexure, hepatic flexure, and cecum
    b. Mucosal pattern assessable on postevacuation film
    c. Distensibility and contractility indicative of wall pliability

13. Gastrointestinal studies useful indicator of abnormality because of close apposition to bony pelvis, spine, liver, pancreas, aorta, retroperitoneal nodes, kidneys

IV. Lymphatic system and spleen
   A. Lymph node groups
      1. Parietal—behind peritoneum, adjoining larger blood vessels
      2. Visceral—related to visceral arteries
      3. Parameters
         a. Density—soft tissue usual
            (1) Calcifications—infection or tumor

(2) Artificially increased (lymphangiography)
    b. Size—increased
       (1) Soft tissue mass
       (2) May displace adjoining structures, such as kidney, ureter, bladder, gastrointestinal tract
    c. Contour
       (1) Difficult to assess without contrast media
       (2) Lobulation of value in differential diagnosis
  B. Spleen—(parameters)
     1. Contour and margination
        a. Sharpness of outline dependent on condition of surrounding tissue
        b. Alteration in sharpness and contour may effect adjoining structures (stomach margin in perisplenitis)
     2. Size
        a. Increased
           (1) Displacing adjoining structures
           (2) Roentgenography occasionally only way of detecting
           (3) Reflects infiltration, hyperactivity, congestion, primary cyst or tumor
        b. Absent—congenital or postsurgical
     3. Location—may be displaced by adjoining structures (e.g., pancreatic mass)
     4. Number—may have accessory spleens

V. Urinary system
   A. Components
      1. Excretory—kidney parenchyma
      2. Collecting—collecting tubules, calyces, renal pelvis, ureters, bladder
      3. Expulsive—bladder, bladder neck, urethra
   B. Density
      1. Naturally occurring
         a. Soft tissue density
         b. Fat (radiolucent)—perirenal, renal sinus
      2. Naturally occuring—increased
         a. (Calcification) calculus—form and number may indicate etiology and type
         b. Tumor—pattern clue to type of tumor
         c. Vascular
            (1) Usually arterial
            (2) Occasionally in angioma
            (3) May outline aneurysm
         d. Postinflammatory
      3. Naturally occurring—decreased
         a. Excess fat renal sinus
         b. Adjoining lipoma
      4. Artifically increased
         a. Intravenous injection and renal excretion (intravenous pyelogram)—usual method
            (1) Films taken shortly after injection for density of kidney from excretion of medium

        (2) Uniformity of parenchymal opacification and rate of excretion seen

        (3) Subsequent films—opacification of internal aspect of collecting structures develops

    b. Direct injection—increased density

        (1) Percutaneous into cyst

        (2) Catheters into bladder and ureters (retrograde pyelography)

C. Contour

  1. Kidney

    a. Outlined by perirenal fat

    b. Usually smooth margin with hilum identifiable

    c. Central hump left kidney—"dromedary kidney" from splenic pressure

    d. Lobulated

        (1) Excess tissue in or adjacent to kidney

        (2) Cyst, tumor, carbuncle may cause

        (3) Persistance of fetal lobulation—uncommon

    e. Irregular cortex—scarring from infection or infarction

  2. Collecting structures

    a. Deformed by adjoining structures: lymph nodes, retroperitoneal masses, aberrant vessels, dilated periureteric arteries or veins, uterus, prostate

    b. Intrinsic deformity

        (1) Narrow and irregular—scarring from trauma or infection

        (2) Narrow—spasm—transient

        (3) Wall irregular from tumor deposit

        (4) Protrusion of wall—diverticulum—usually bladder

D. Size

  1. Kidney—tables of normal available

    a. Enlarged—generalized

        (1) Hypertrophy parenchyma—compensatory hypertrophy

        (2) Hydronephrosis—dilatation of collecting structures

        (3) Unusual tissue infiltrate—tumor, fluid (edema)

    b. Enlarged—focal (lobulated)—cyst, tumor, carbuncle

    c. Small

        (1) Congenital hypoplasia

        (2) Atrophy

           (a) Postinflammatory

           (b) Decreased blood flow

  2. Collecting structures

    a. Enlarged

        (1) Obstruction to flow of urine

        (2) Atony—neurologic deficit or lack of stimulus (neurogenic bladder)

    b. Small

        (1) Compression by adjoining structures

        (2) Peripheral scarring—postinflammatory, retroperitoneal fibrosis, postradiation effect urinary bladder

E. Location

  1. Kidney

    a. Left usually higher than right

    b. Lower pole anteriorly placed compared to upper pole

    c. Normally descend in erect position unless fixed by adjoining abnormality

    d. Easily displaced by adjoining masses

    e. Upward migration right kidney with cirrhosis liver

  2. Collecting structures

    a. Ureteral displacement common with retroperitoneal masses

    b. Bladder displaced by intrapelvic masses

    c. Renal pelvis displaced by parapelvic excess tissue (parapelvic cyst)

F. Number

  1. Kidney

    a. Rare—accessory kidney

    b. Fusion right and left kidney producing only one kidney (horseshoe kidney)

    c. One absent—congenital or postsurgical

  2. Collecting structures

    a. Duplication calyces, ureters, pelves—common

    b. Duplication partial or complete

    c. Postsurgical absence

G. Margination

  1. Kidney

    a. Sharpness dependent on status perirenal fat

    b. Decrease in edema, fibrosis or inanition

  2. Collecting structures

    a. Only bladder shown without use of contrast media

    b. External wall bladder difficult to see without good intrapelvic fat deposits

VI. Reproductive system

  A. Components (demonstrable roentgenographically)

    1. Ovary

    2. Uterus

    3. Vagina

    4. Fallopian tubes

    5. Prostate

    6. Seminal vesicles

    7. External genitalia

  B. Density

    1. Naturally occurring—usual—soft tissue

    2. Naturally occurring—increased—calcification

      a. Prostatic—common—small—retropubic

      b. Uterus—frequent

        (1) Usually fibromyomata—non-pregnant

        (2) Fetal skeleton—after fourth month of gestation

      c. Ovary—tumor, cyst, old infection

        (1) Type of calcification clue to nature of lesion—psammomatous calcification fibroma

        (2) Teeth within dermoid

      d. Fallopian tubes and seminal vesicles

        (1) Inflammation—old

        (2) Usually linear

        (3) Resembles arterial wall calcification

3. Naturally occurring—reduced—fatty tumor—ovarian dermoid
4. Artificially increased
   a. Vagina, uterine cavity, fallopian tubes (hysterosalpingography)
      (1) Iodinated medium injected into cervical canal
      (2) Outlines internal configuration—retrograde
      (3) Passage into peritoneal cavity—fallopian tubes patent
5. Artifically reduced (around intraperitoneal structures)
   a. Gas into peritoneal cavity (gynecogram)
   b. Delineates location, number, size ovaries, uterus

C. Size
   1. Uterus
      a. Enlarged
         (1) Intrapelvic soft tissue mass
         (2) Adjoining organs displaced—may require contrast studies to show, e.g., barium enema
         (3) Pregnancy most frequent cause
         (4) Lobulated—usually tumor
      b. Small
         (1) Infantile uterus
         (2) Usually not seen without gynecogram
         (3) Surgical absence—frequent
   2. Ovaries
      a. Enlarged
         (1) Soft tissue mass—lateral or central pelvic space and lower abdomen
         (2) May rise out of pelvis
         (3) Displacement adjoining organs (colon, small bowel) frequent
         (4) Incorporated in inflammatory mass (tubovarian abscess)
         (5) Stein-Leventhal syndrome (requires gynecogram to show)
      b. Small
         (1) Hypoplasia—congenital
         (2) Surgical absence
   3. Prostate—enlarged—only size change demonstrable on routine contrast study
      a. Elevates base of urinary bladder
      b. Narrows prostatic urethra
      c. Requires contrast study urinary tract to demonstrate
   4. Vagina
      a. Absent or small—intersex
      b. Vaginogram—opaque material in vagina—required to assess
      c. Postinflammatory or post-radiation scarring—may be shown by filling through fistula from bladder or colon

D. Location
   1. Uterus
      a. Retroflexed—may press on rectum
      b. Anteflexed—pressure on urinary bladder on urography
   2. Ovaries
      a. Displaced by adjoining masses (requires gynecogram)
      b. Ectopia—unusual location
      c. Retracted—scarring from inflammation

The naturally occurring contrast between the structures of the chest facilitates radiographic examination of this area. While certain structures, such as the esophagus and the internal structures of the heart, must be artificially changed in density for complete study, the bulk of radiographic diagnostic procedures of the chest can be accomplished by using only the natural contrast. The abdomen, on the other hand, contains several structures that have similar radiographic densities (Fig. 2-1): the liver, pancreas, spleen, kidneys, muscles, and the fluid-filled intestinal tract. When one observes a film of the abdomen which is uniform in density, as seen in Fig. 2-2, it becomes apparent that even the minor normal contrasts can be obliterated by other substances; in this instance, ascites or excess intra-abdominal fluid has obscured the fat lines normally identifiable. As a result, many of the special examinations routinely used in diagnostic roentgenography are designed to induce artificial contrast change in abdominal structures. The gastrointestinal series, barium enema, pneumocolon, and small bowel studies are all designed to outline the intestinal tract (Figs. 2-3 to 2-6). Oral cholecystography, intravenous cholangiography, transhepatic cholangiography, operative and postoperative cholangiography, hepatography, and splenoportography have all been developed to produce opacification of usually nonopaque organs (Figs.

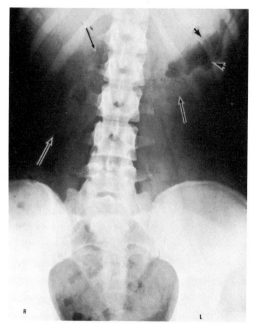

Fig. 2-1. The radiolucency of retroperitoneal fat and gas, contrasted against the water density of the soft tissue structures in the abdomen, makes the demonstration of organs possible. The long solid arrows point to the poles of the kidneys which rest on the oblique lines of the psoas margins. Immediately above the right kidney is the adrenal gland. The soft tissue density in the right upper quadrant is the liver. Gas lies within the lumen of the stomach (open arrows on the left side of the abdomen). The radiolucent gas within the colon and small bowel is present in many areas in the abdomen.

2-7 to 2-10). Various forms of urography (Figs. 2-11 to 2-13), retroperitoneal pneumography, and intra-abdominal gynecography induce either increased or decreased contrast to outline the anatomic structures and demonstrate their ability to function. Even structures, such as the lumbar spine, that have a high degree of natural contrast require additional artificially induced contrast to allow complete study. In this way, study of the intraspinal structures is possible through myelography. In consideration of the abdomen, as in the chest, an organized evaluation of the organ systems incorporated in that area must be made. Therefore, myelography fits, in part, in the category of abdominal studies.

The interrelationship of abnormalities among the various systems must be searched for. If abnormal calcium deposits are present in the region of the kidneys and the bones generally appear somewhat less calcified than normal, diseases such as hyperparathyroidism should be considered (Fig. 2-14). Detailed study of the various systems demonstrated on the film of the abdomen may lead to a definitive diagnosis that would otherwise be obscured. The component systems to be considered are: (1) musculoskeletal, (2) gastrointestinal, (3) hepatopancreatic, (4) lymphatic and spleen, and (5) genitourinary. Films of the abdomen also often show the lower portions of the lungs and the diaphragmatic leaves; these have been discussed in Chapter 1. The vascular system is represented by the abdominal aorta, portal system, inferior vena cava, renovascular complex, and the diffuse vessels of the intestinal tract (see Fig. 2-13).

Text continued on p. 89.

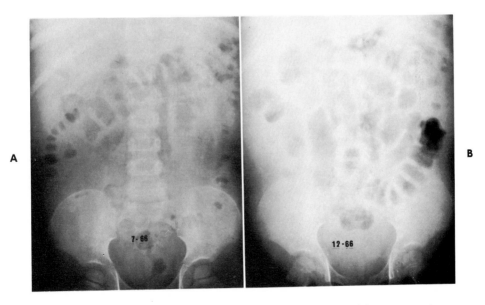

Fig. 2-2. A, Excess fluid in the abdomen (ascites) produces a general haziness on the roentgenograms. The distribution of the gas of the bowel is, however, reasonably normal although the psoas margins are obscured. **B,** Six months later the fluid has increased and the gas filled loops of bowel are now seen to be separated from the lateral wall of the abdomen; they have floated upward on the fluid with the patient lying on her back. In this instance, it is the result of nephrosis in a child.

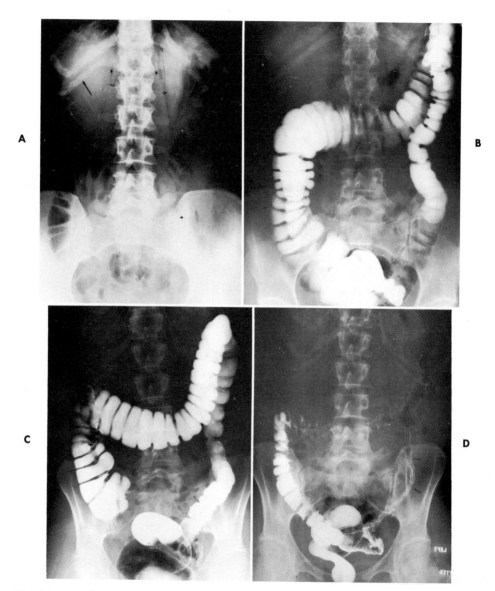

Fig. 2-3. **A,** Preliminary plain film of the abdomen before a barium enema shows the psoas margins and renal outlines (open arrows). Normal variations in the skeletal system are noted. The short solid arrows in the upper abdomen point to the articulation at the base of lumbar ribs. The lower solid arrow indicates a transitional vertebra, one that resembles the sacrum on one side. The long solid arrows in the upper quadrants show extensively calcified costal cartilages which may be mistaken for intra-abdominal calcifications. The amount of gas present in the colon is normal in an individual who has taken laxatives and enemas in preparation for the examination. **B,** The alteration of location of the barium and air between the P-A (**C**) and the A-P (**B**) projections shows the effect of gravity. **C,** The small solid arrow indicates the normal appearing haustral pattern. The open arrow is the point of peritoneal reflection between the descending and sigmoid colon segments. **D,** The mucosal pattern (solid arrows), which may normally be somewhat linear, is shown.

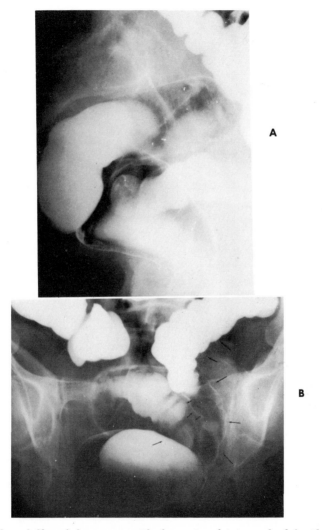

Fig. 2-4. A, The lateral film of the rectum with the patient lying on the left side shows the distensibility of the colon and the rectum, with good demonstration of the walls of the rectum. **B,** A special projection (Chassard-Lapine), used to uncoil the loops of the sigmoid colon. The haustral pattern is identifiable (small solid arrows).

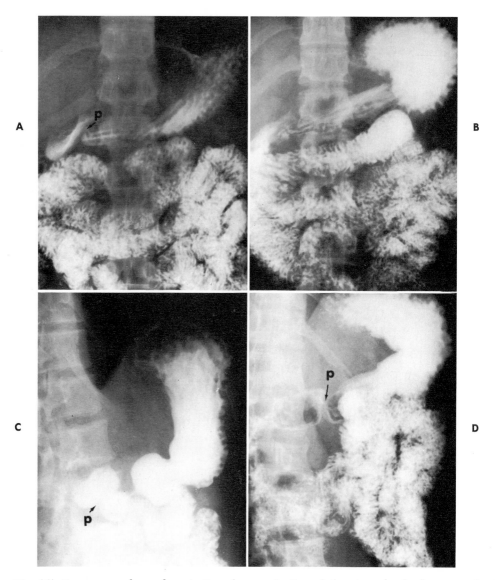

Fig. 2-5. Four commonly used projections for examination of the stomach, duodenum, and proximal small bowel are the P-A (**A**), A-P (**B**), right anterior oblique (**C**), and left posterior oblique (**D**). The gas in the stomach migrates to the uppermost portion; therefore, in the P-A projection the fundus contains gas, whereas in the A-P projection gas lies in the antrum and duodenal bulb. In the right anterior oblique projection, gas lies in the fundus; in the left posterior oblique gas lies in the antrum and the duodenal bulb. The pylorus (*p*) is best seen in the oblique projection with the duodenal bulb lying just beyond the canal and the gastric antrum just proximal thereto. This is a normal study.

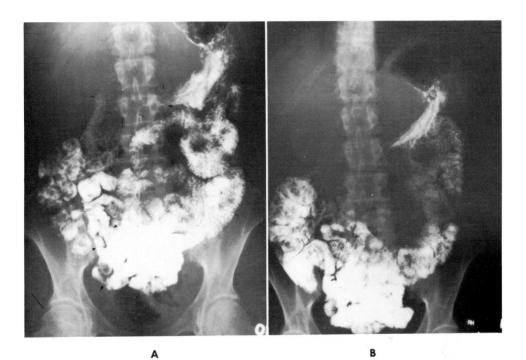

A   **B**

Fig. 2-6. A, A film taken 30 minutes after the patient has drunk barium shows the distribution of barium along the course of the small bowel. The small arrows in the upper abdomen show the mucosal pattern of the duodenum, the open arrow in the central portion of the abdomen shows the jejunum, and the lower solid arrows show the ileum. This is a normal pattern. **B,** A film made 30 minutes later shows the barium in the ascending colon and distal ileum. The ileocecal valve is identified (small solid arrows). Of incidental interest is the degenerative change observed in the region of the right hip joint (**A**). The width of the bowel wall is shown in the right lower quadrant (opposing open arrows).

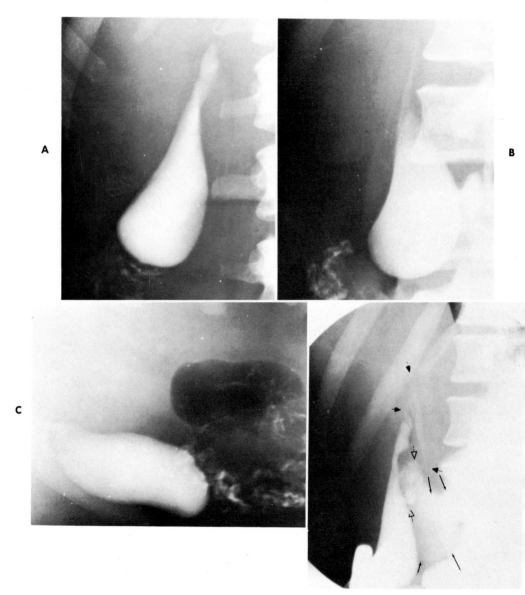

Fig. 2-7. A, P-A prone and **B,** left anterior oblique prone films obtained after the patient had ingested iodinated compounds show the outline of the gallbladder. **C,** With the patient lying on the right side the gallbladder shows a change in form. If stones were present within the gallbladder these would usually settle to the dependent portion. **D,** After a fatty meal a normal gallbladder usually contracts. The cystic duct with the valves of Heister, the hepatic duct (upper solid arrows) and the common duct (lower solid arrow) are opacified when the iodinated bile is forced from the gallbladder. The duodenal bulb (open arrows) and the antrum of the stomach (small solid arrows) are opacified by barium remaining after a gastrointestinal series. The relationship of the gallbladder, duodenal bulb, antrum of the stomach, and hepatic flexure of the colon can be identified.

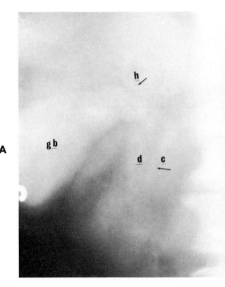

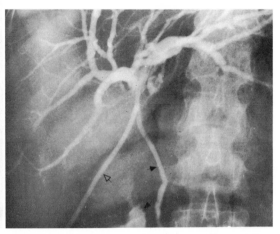

A

gb

h

d   c

Fig. 2-8. **A,** Better opacification of the biliary ductal system may result from intravenous injection of an iodinated compound. This is a tomographic cut of a normal intravenous cholangiogram. The gallbladder (*gb*) is opacified, as are the hepatic duct (*h*) and the common duct (*c*). The common duct is beginning to taper as it reaches the level of the ampulla of Vater. From here the iodinated compound enters the duodenum (*d*). **B,** Percutaneous cholangiography (opacification of the biliary ducts by direct injection of iodinated material through a catheter [open arrow] passed into the hepatic duct through the skin) allows good visualization of the biliary ducts. The common duct (upper solid arrow) is small as the result of scarring, but the contrast medium is seen to enter the duodenum (lower solid arrow).

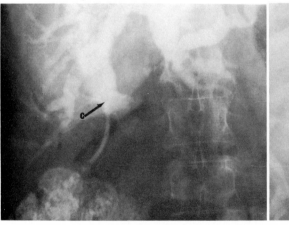

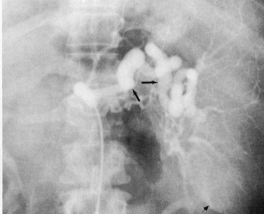

Fig. 2-9. **A,** At the time of surgery, catheters can be placed into the common duct (*C*, arrow) and opacification of the biliary tree accomplished to show obstruction. The width of the biliary ducts in this instance is quite great, indicative of prolonged obstruction. **B,** Injection of an iodinated compound through a catheter placed in the splenic vein enables visualization of the upper abdominal viscera. The splenic vein (long solid arrows) is quite tortuous. The spleen (small solid arrow) also opacifies. As the result of increased pressure, the contrast medium does not enter the portal system. In this instance it represents congenital portal hypertension. Some opacification is occurring in the vessels of the fundus of the stomach in the upper portion of the picture.

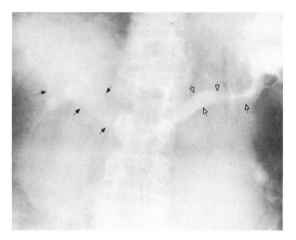

Fig. 2-10. By placement of a needle into the spleen and injection of an iodinated compound directly into it, opacification can also be obtained of the splenic vein (open arrows) and, in this instance, the portal vein (solid arrows). This is a splenoportogram.

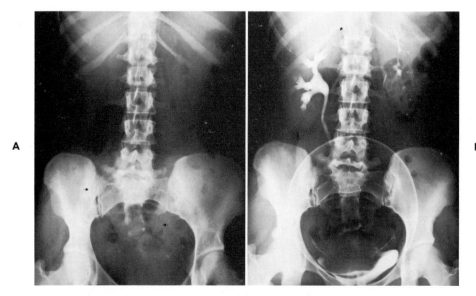

Fig. 2-11. Evaluation of the function and anatomy of the kidneys can be accomplished by intravenous injection of an iodinated compound (intravenous pyelogram). **A,** An initial film is taken to determine abnormal densities and the form of the structures. In this instance the sacrum is scoliotic and there is stress response about the margins of the sacroiliac joints (solid arrows). This is only a coincidental finding. **B,** Five minutes after the injection there is good concentration of the medium in both kidneys, and the collecting structures are well seen. The upper and lower poles of the right kidney are identifiable (solid arrows). The rounded density overlying the lower abdomen is a compression device to partially obstruct the ureters, thereby better defining the upper portion of the urinary tract. It is quite effective, in this instance, on the right side but not as effective on the left.

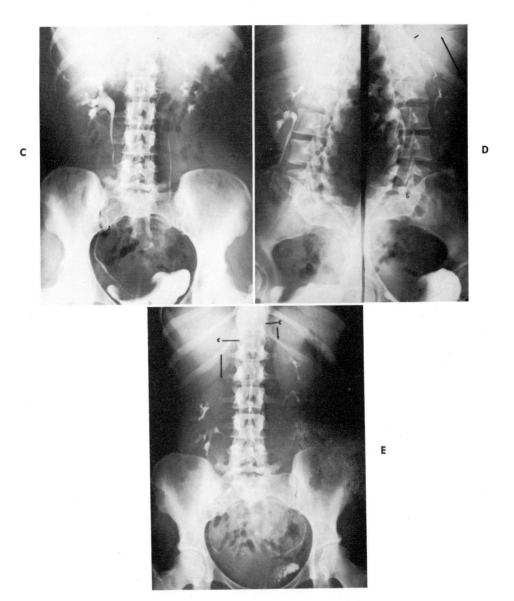

Fig. 2-11, cont'd. C, At the end of 10 minutes the compression device is removed and it can be seen that the opacified urine is draining from the right side. The superior margin of the bladder is deformed (open arrow) because of pressure from the adjoining uterus. **D**, Oblique views taken at the same time show that the longitudinal axis of the kidneys (solid line) runs at an angle to the spine and parallels the psoas margin (upper open arrow). The upper pole of the left kidney is indicated by the short line. Of incidental interest is a spondylolysis of L5 on the left (open arrow). **E**, At the end of 20 minutes with the patient erect the bladder has emptied as a result of the patient's voiding. Good drainage of the opacified urine from the kidneys is now seen. As the result of the erect position both kidneys have descended from the position observed in **B** (*C*, original level of upper poles—arrows show amount of descent). This is a normal finding. Changes in density and position, therefore, are both used in evaluating normality of the renal structure.

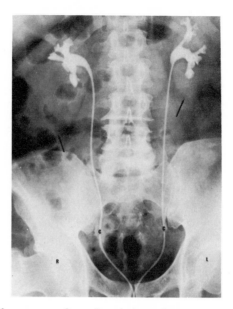

Fig. 2-12. Instillation of opaque medium directly into the urinary tract can be accomplished by placing catheters (*C*) through the bladder, up the ureters, and into the renal pelves. The outlines of the kidneys are seen (solid arrows) and the internal structures are identifiable after injection of iodinated compound. The kidney on the left is normal. The one on the right is enlarged and there is deformity of the internal structure. This alteration in form is the result of a large cyst at the lower pole of the right kidney.

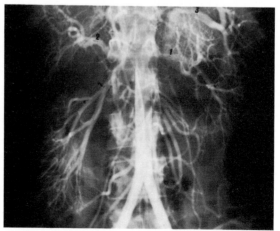

Fig. 2-13. Another way to change density artificially is to introduce a catheter along the femoral artery into the aorta and inject an iodinated compound. In this instance the renal arteries (*1*) are well seen with opacification of the renal parenchyma. The celiac axis and the inferior mesenteric and superior mesenteric arteries are identifiable, as are the hepatic artery (*2*) and splenic artery (*3*). This type of examination is very valuable for assessing abnormalities of the renal structures, particularly in cases of tumor.

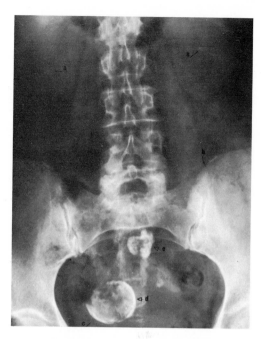

Fig. 2-14. Naturally occurring variations in densities are illustrated in this roentgenogram of an individual suffering from a parathyroid adenoma. As the result of hyperparathyroidism, renal calculi (*a*) have formed bilaterally. There is resorption of the bony structure along the medial aspect of the iliac crest (*b*), and the general density of the osseous structures as a whole is somewhat reduced. Coincidental calcification has occurred in a large uterine fibroid (*d,* open arrow), which is set off from the urinary bladder by a line of fat (*c*). Calcific deposits have also occurred in the presacral lymph nodes (*e,* open arrow).

Musculoskeletal system

The structures of the musculoskeletal system usually identifiable on the films of the abdomen include the lumbar spine, pelvis, hip joints, proximal femora, lower ribs, thoracolumbar spine, sacrum, coccyx, sacroiliac articulations, and occasionally, if the arms are at the side, the bony components of the hands and wrists. The properitoneal fat lines, the diaphragmatic leaves, and the gluteal masses are all common landmarks in assessing the soft tissues of the abdomen.

In careful evaluation of the lumbar spine and pelvis, the bony components and the alignment of the vertebral bodies are easily discernible. The usual projection of the abdomen is taken with the patient lying on his back with the beam entering from above and recording on the film behind the patient. Only side-to-side misalignments, usually in the form of a scoliosis, can be demonstrated with this projection. The significance of the misalignment depends upon the degree of the curve, how many vertebrae are involved in the curve, and whether the pelvis also shows the effect of such a curve. Scoliosis can be a manifestation of many conditions, such as muscle spasm, paralysis, idiopathic, abnormal form of the vertebrae, unequal leg length, or diseases of the lower extremities (Fig. 2-15). The bony pelvis reflects long-standing abnormal alignments in that the sacrum

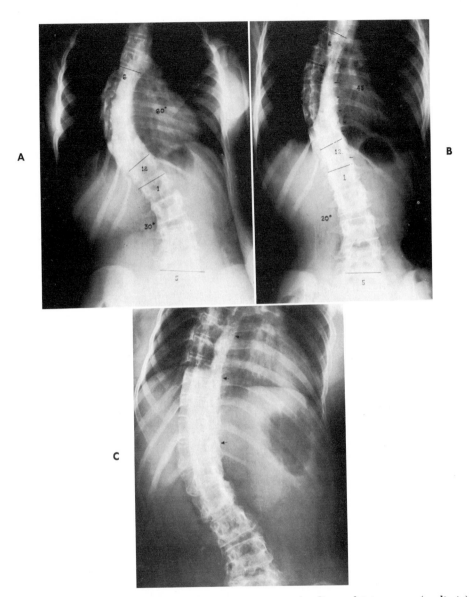

Fig. 2-15. Alignment of the thoracic and lumbar spine may be distorted into curves (scoliosis).
A, Idiopathic scoliosis occurs in late childhood or early adolescence and is more frequent in
females. The degree of curve can be measured by using landmarks, in this instance, superior
margins of the pedicles of the sixth thoracic and twelfth thoracic vertebrae and the superior
margin of the pedicles of the first and fifth lumbar vertebrae. The superior angle measures
60° and the inferior angle 30°. B, Following posterior fusion a fusion mass is identifiable along
the concavity of the scoliosis (small solid arrows). It is observed that as the result of corrective
measures thoracic scoliosis has been reduced to 45° and the lumbar 20°. C, The type of
curve resulting from poliomyelitis with paralysis is a long C shaped scoliosis. Again a posterior
fusion has produced a bony mass (solid arrows). This is aimed at stabilizing the spine. The
ribs have also shown deformity; the right ribs project less laterally and those on the left project more laterally and are elongated in adaptive response to the scoliosis.

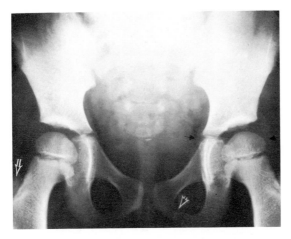

Fig. 2-16. The film of the abdomen usually includes the pelvis; its appearance varies with age. This is a normal film for a 5-year-old child. The middle arrow indicates the appearance of the incompletely ossified Y cartilage of the acetabulum. The secondary ossification centers for the head of the femur are seen on either side (outer solid arrow). Visible at the edges of the film are the ossification centers for the greater trochanter (outlined arrow). The junction of the pubis and the ischium in the region of the obturator foramen is irregular (open arrow), a normal finding for one of this age. Lateral to the hip joints are soft tissue densities that represent the normal configuration of the capsule of the hip joint.

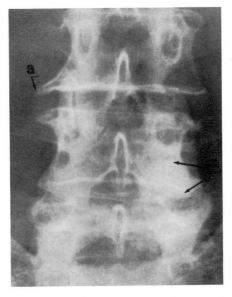

Fig. 2-17. There has been a change in the size, configuration, and density of the bony structures of the lumbar spine. Hypertrophic spur formation (*a*) is the result of both degeneration and excess bulging of the intervertebral disc. There is excess bone deposit (*b*) about the apophysial joints posteriorly, again the result of degeneration. In contrast to the scoliosis the alignment of the components of the spine is not greatly altered. Prolonged scoliosis may, however, predispose to degenerative change such as this.

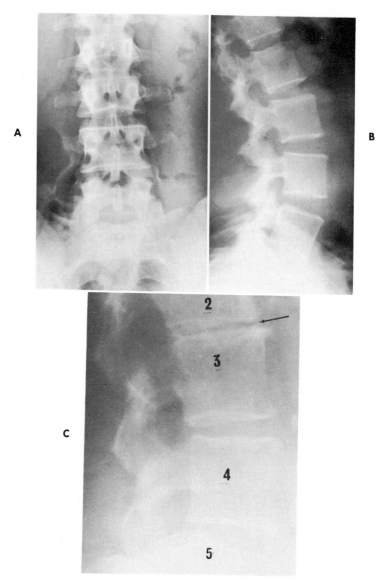

Fig. 2-18. The normal configuration of the vertebral bodies is illustrated. **A,** In this projection there may be a minor scoliosis, which is considered normal. **B,** In the lateral projection with the patient standing, there is an anterior curvature (lordosis) with some narrowing of the posterior portion of the intervertebral disc as compared to the anterior portion. This is a normal phenomenon. **C,** In contrast to the normal spine, the intervertebral disc between the second and third lumbar vertebrae is severely narrowed. The arrow points to gas that has formed in the anterior aspect of the disc; this is pathognomonic of degenerative disc disease. In addition, the intervertebral disc between the third and fourth lumbar vertebrae is narrow. As the result the margins of the vertebrae are more parallel than between the fourth and fifth lumbar vertebrae, another sign of loss of substance of the intervertebral disc. The bones are less dense because of osteoporosis as the result of treatment with steroids.

also shows a scoliosis. The developmental pattern of the pelvis should be recognized (Fig. 2-16).

The contour of the individual vertebrae, pelvis, and sacrum reflects abnormal pressure such as scoliosis. Focal disease also produces an abnormality of contour that may relate to overgrowth but is much more frequently manifested by decreased or irregular size. Among the most common causes of an abnormal contour resulting from overgrowth is hypertrophic response to degenerative change. This is seen as "spur" formation. Advanced hypertrophic spurring is shown in Fig. 2-17. Frequently, the vertebrae at the same level will have decreased vertical dimension as a result of compression. The size and contour of the intervertebral discs should also be studied. These discs normally increase in vertical dimension from the upper to the lower portions of the spine. The disc between the last lumbar vertebra and the first sacral vertebra, however, may normally be somewhat less in its vertical dimension. The normal curves of the spine, that is, anterior bowing in the cervical and lumbar spine and posterior bowing in the thoracic area, produce a corresponding change in the configuration of the intervertebral discs. In the lumbar region, the height of the disc is normally greater anteriorly than posteriorly (Fig. 2-18). If the margins of the discs in the lumbar spine are parallel when the patient is erect, however, one must be suspicious of degenerative change of the intervertebral disc. It is essential to understand the anatomy of the spine as seen on the roentgenograms (Fig. 2-19). Long-standing malalignment will produce a wedging of the vertebrae with one margin shorter than the other. Contour is also a most sensitive indicator of developmental abnormalities of the spine. These abnormalities include hemivertebrae, in which only half of each vertebra forms (Fig. 2-20); spina bifida, in which the posterior part of the neural arch fails to unite; and transitional vertebrae (Fig. 2-21), in which the vertebrae more closely resemble the adjoining area than a true lumbar-type vertebra. Other severe anomalies may occur (Fig. 2-22).

Inflammation and fracture also alter the appearance of the vertebrae and usually cause some loss in the expected height of the vertebrae (Fig. 2-23).

The number of the vertebrae may vary from one individual to another. Normally, there are five lumbar segments, five sacral segments, and three coccygeal segments. An excess number of lumbar segments may result from lumbarization of the first sacral segment. The coccyx and sacrum are the most frequent sites of excess segmentation.

Having evaluated the number, contour, and alignment of the spinal segments demonstrated on the abdominal film, one should then assess the density of the bony structures. Normally, the relative density of the lumbar spine and pelvis should be similar, since they are both part of the axial skeleton. The use of naturally occurring densities as indicators of disease or normality is a fairly crude method since it has been shown that 40% of any vertebral body must be removed before the defect can be shown roentgenographically. Thus, before definite decreased mineralization of the osseous structures can be demonstrated, rather severe bone loss has occurred. The most common cause for decreased mineralization and density is osteoporosis of old age. Inflammation, metastatic tumor de-

Text continued on p. 100.

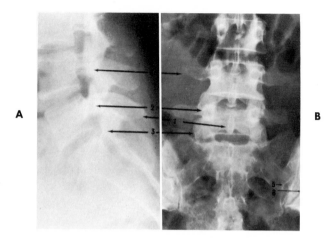

Fig. 2-19. Films may be taken of the lumbosacral area specifically. The anatomy identifiable in this normal study shows the spinous processes (*1*) as seen on the lateral (**A**) and and A-P (**B**) projection. The pedicles (*2*) and superior facets (*3*) of S1 and the transverse processes (*4*) can be identified in both projections. The posterior margin (*5*) and the anterior aspect (*6*) of the sacroiliac joint are seen. Their sharpness and alignment indicate normality.

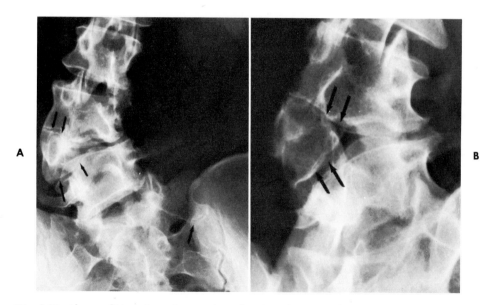

Fig. 2-20. Abnormalities of number, such as hemivertebra or malsegmentation, are frequent. **A,** In this instance, the fourth lumbar vertebra is a hemivertebra, with the body in the A-P projection being outlined with arrows. Note that the pedicle and transverse process are present on this side. With the most frequent form of hemivertebra there is a complete posterior and anterior set of structures on one side and complete absence on the other. The lower arrow indicates the transitional state of what would appear to be the first sacral vertebra. **B,** In the oblique projection the body of the hemivertebra lies posteriorly as compared to the adjoining vertebrae.

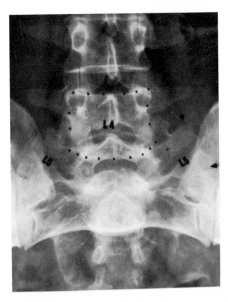

Fig. 2-21. Occasionally transitional vertebrae at the lumbosacral junction show bilateral articulations with the sacral wing. The transverse processes of the fifth lumbar vertebra (L5) are quite broad as outlined by arrows. The sacrum has a very horizontally placed curve so that the body of the fourth lumbar vertebra (L4), as outlined by dots, is on an angle and not well seen. In this instance, alteration of both form and alignment indicates the nature of the abnormality.

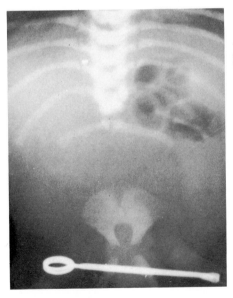

Fig. 2-22. Severe anomalies of the lumbar spine may occur. In this infant, there is change in form, alignment, number, and density in that there has been failure of development of the entire lumbar spine and sacrum and absence of the major portion of the body of the twelfth thoracic vertebra. In spite of the severe anomaly there is evidence of neurologic function in the lower extremities upon examination of the patient. The metallic density overlying the pelvis is a clamp which is placed on the umbilical cord after birth.

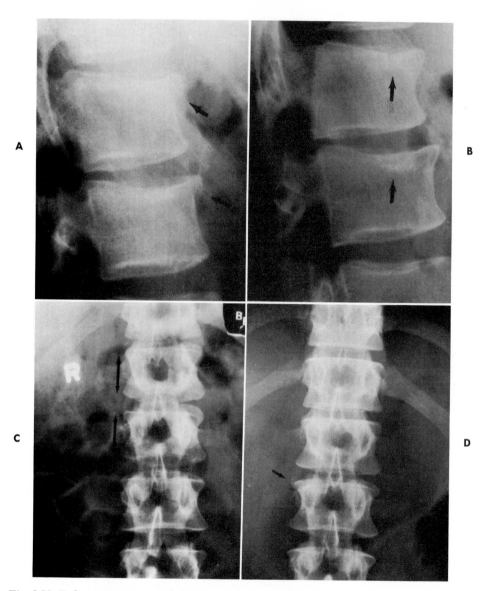

Fig. 2-23. Deformity consisting of change of form and density may result from trauma. **A,** An acute flexion injury has produced compression fractures of the anterior superior margins of the bodies of the first and second lumbar vertebrae (arrows). **B,** Fourteen months later the major portion of the fracture has healed; however, the intervertebral discs have penetrated into the vertebral bodies (arrows), and there has been loss of the normal height of the intervertebral discs. **C,** In the A-P projection a loss of vertical dimension of the right side of the vertebral bodies of the first and second lumbar vertebrae is observed (arrows). **D,** Fourteen months later a spur (arrow) has formed along the right side of the body of the second lumbar vertebra, showing the result of healing trauma and disc protrusion.

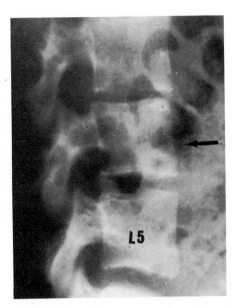

Fig. 2-24. Bone density and form in the lumbar spine is changed by infection. Shortly after the onset of retroperitoneal inflammatory disease the body of L4 shows some minor loss of substance anteriorly, indicated by the solid arrow.

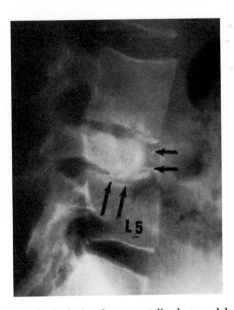

Fig. 2-25. Seven months later the body has been partially destroyed but is encased in density as the result of new bone formation. The disc between L4 and L5 has been destroyed, and irregular areas of bone deposit as well as depression of the superior margin of the body of L5 are indicated (solid arrows).

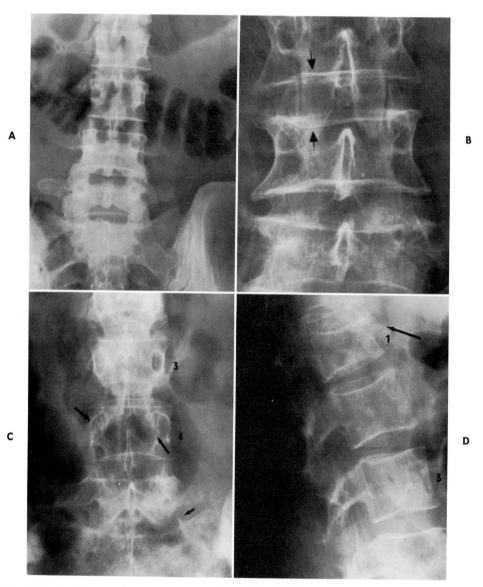

Fig. 2-26. A, The normal texture and configuration of the lumbar spine is shown. B, Osteoporosis is present and manifested by the coarse trabecular pattern and loss of calcium content, with preservation of cortical margins and minor intrusion of the intervertebral disc into the vertebral bodies (solid arrows). C, Metastatic disease from carcinoma of the breast is demonstrated, showing loss of the right pedicle of L4 (top arrow), loss of substance of the lamina on the left at L4 (middle arrow), and the region of the sacrum on the left at L5-S1 (lower arrow). D, The compression and fragmentation of the anterior aspect of the body of L1 is seen on the lateral projection (arrow).

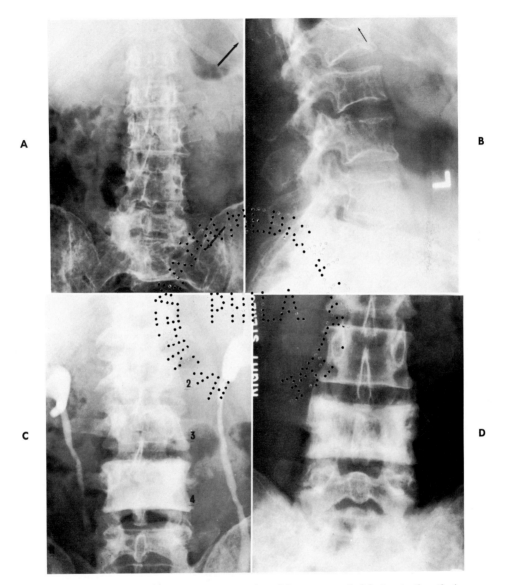

Fig. 2-27. **A,** Multiple myeloma as seen is manifested by an expanded lesion in the rib (upper arrow), diffuse loss of bone substance, and focal loss of bone substance in the left wing of the sacrum (lower arrow). **B,** In the lateral projection the vertebral bodies are compressed both from above and below; this compression involves both the anterior and the posterior aspects of the vertebrae, showing total loss of support. There is a disordered pattern to the trabeculae. **C,** Lymphoma and carcinoma of the prostate may induce dense osteoblastic response as shown. **D,** This is in contrast to the appearance of Paget's disease where the vertebral body is enlarged and there is dense trabecular pattern with the major density around the periphery of the margins. This produces a picture-frame type of vertebra. The pedicles, laminae, and sacrum are also involved.

posits, primary bone tumors, lack of adequate calcium, or endocrinopathies may also remove calcium or prevent its deposit in the bone (Figs. 2-24 to 2-27). Whether the demineralization is focal or generalized becomes an important clue to the cause of the calcium loss. The vertebral bodies are more severely involved with osteoporosis. There is also a loss of mineralization of the pedicles, neural arches, spinous processes, and transverse processes, but the rather small amount of medullary bone and greater amount of cortical bone mask the osteoporosis. The fact that the posterior elements are frequently involved by metastatic disease provides a clue in distinguishing bony abnormality of metastatic disease from metabolic disease.

The lumbar spine is one of the most common sites of osseous metastatic deposits. Since heavy venous channels surround the vertebrae, run through the spinal canal, and penetrate the vertebrae, tumor deposits filtered out of the bloodstream give rise to metastatic disease.

Healing fractures, healing of inflammation, degeneration of the intervertebral discs with sclerosis of the adjoining vertebrae, metastatic tumors, primarily prostate or lymphoma, or excess bone deposits as in Paget's disease all produce increased density of the bone. Full understanding of the significance of increased density requires understanding of the formation of bone. Numerous excellent works are available describing this entire process. One of these is *Fundamentals of Roentgenology* by L. F. Squire.

The intraspinal contents comprise the meninges, spinal cord, vessels, and nerve roots. Artificially changed contrast (myelography) is required to outline these structures. In myelography a needle is inserted and a contrast medium is injected into the subarachnoid space, usually between the third and fourth or fourth and fifth lumbar segments (Fig. 2-28). Since elemental iodine has a high potential for absorbing radiation, iodinated compounds are commonly used. Air may also serve as a contrast substance. The medium used in the United States is oily and heavier than the cerebrospinal fluid and is not resorbed easily by the body. The material used in some European countries is water-soluble and resorbable. Myelography can be compared to the examination of a water filled hose with rather fixed curves into which a quantity of mercury is placed. The study of the inside of the hose is accomplished by tilting the hose in such a way that the mercury opacifies segments of the hose. Abnormalities pushing on the hose change the appearance of the mercury column. Unusual material within the hose causes the mercury column to split or prevents the column from flowing into certain segments. The spinal cord, which normally lies within the canal, and the nerve roots extending from the termination of the cord to the lumbar segments have a predictable appearance, and changes in this appearance indicate abnormalities. Usually, there is some opacification of the short arachnoidal pouches which continue along the nerve roots in the region of the neural foramina. The failure of these "nerve root cuffs" to fill results from abnormal pressure on the cuffs or obstruction to the flow of the contrast medium as a result of scarring. The most common intrinsic cause for such obstruction is fibrosis caused by inflammation or degeneration. Extrinsic pressure in most cases represents a

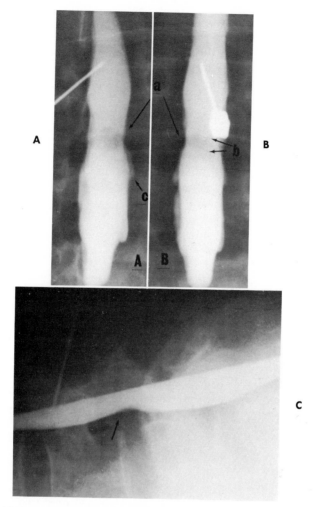

Fig. 2-28. A, Oblique projection: the subarachnoid space is opacified by introduction of an iodinated oily medium through a lumbar puncture needle (myelography). **B,** Prone A-P: a somewhat different form of the contrast column is observed. At (*a*) a protruding intervertebral disc causes a marginal deformity and thinning of the contrast column (*b*). The nerve root (*c*) at the next lower level is normal. No nerve root cuff filling is observed at the level of the disc protrusion. **C,** Cross-table lateral projection: with the patient lying prone, it is observed that the contrast column is elevated away from the vertebral bodies (small arrow) by the disc herniation. The degree of elevation indicates that this is a rather markedly herniated nucleus pulposus.

degenerated intervertebral disc with herniation or bony overgrowth around the vertebral bodies. The alignment of the nerve roots may also be altered by adhesion formation or by displacement.

If there is obstruction in the subarachnoid space, the column may not move smoothly as the patient is tilted. Very active pulsations can normally be observed in the cerebrospinal fluid. Lack of such pulsation may indicate an obstruction of the subarachnoid space between the contrast column and the brain.

The intervertebral discs are normally nonopaque. Artificial density may be induced by discography, in which a needle is placed directly into the intervertebral disc and an iodinated compound is injected (Fig. 2-29). Discography demonstrates the intrinsic structure of the disc. If the disc is ruptured, the contrast medium extends beyond the confines of the intervertebral area. Abnormal but naturally occurring alterations in the density of the discs may result from calcification. Degenerative change or acute inflammation in childhood can cause roentgenographic abnormalities. Occasionally, the disc becomes hyperlucent when placed under negative pressure (Fig. 2-30). This is known as the "vacuum disc" phenomenon and results from vaporization of the water within the disc. This phenomenon cannot occur unless a space exists and is positive evidence of degeneration of that disc. Degeneration of the intervertebral disc produces fissuring which creates an abnormal space. It is in this abnormal space that gas collects under negative pressure. The majority of neurologic and neurosurgical spinal disorders which are seen by the physician are related, in part, to disc abnormality.

It must be reemphasized that the vertebral bodies and the intervertebral discs must be studied, but the small posterior joints and transverse processes are to be carefully examined as well. Oblique projections and lateral projections are vital in this study (Fig. 2-31). A common abnormality is spondylolysis, in which there

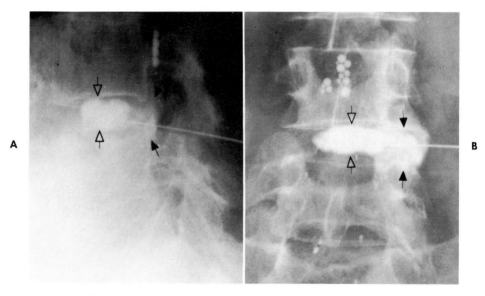

Fig. 2-29. Introduction of contrast medium into the intervertebral disc by a needle placed through the spinal canal (discography). **A,** Lateral projection: the nucleus pulposes (open arrow) which is opacified is lobulated and irregular with posterior escape of the contrast medium (solid arrows) showing rupture of the annulus. Some residual iodophendylate (Pantopaque) is present in the spinal canal from previous myelography. **B,** A-P projection: the nucleus pulposus is better seen (open arrows), but there is lateral and posterior escape of the contrast medium from the annulus fibrosis (solid arrows). This technique enables evaluation of the internal structure of the nucleus and shows the intactness of the annulus fibrosis.

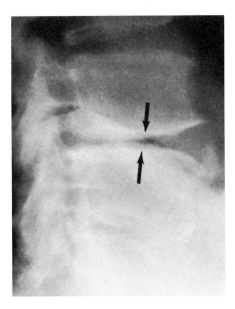

Fig. 2-30. The radiolucent line between the vertebral bodies (solid arrows) represents a vacuum phenomenon. Water vapor forms in the cleft of the degenerated disc as the result of negative pressure created by the body being extended. Spur formation about the anterior aspect of the vertebral bodies indicates degenerative change.

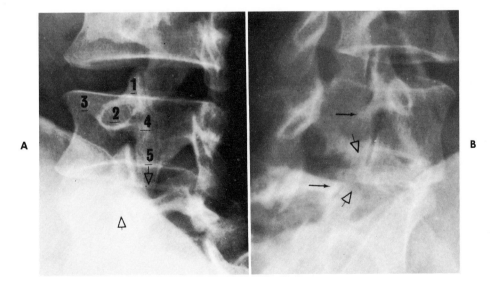

Fig. 2-31. A, Oblique projection of the normal lumbosacral area shows the posterior anatomic structures. These can be thought of as a scotty dog with (*1*) the superior facet (ear), (*2*) the pedicle (eye), (*3*) the transverse process (nose), (*4*) the pars interarticularis (neck), and (*5*) the inferior facet (foreleg). The open arrows show the distance between the inferior facet of L4 and the superior facet of S1. **B,** If spondylolysis is present the pars interarticularis (neck) is broken (small lower arrow) as compared to the normal pars interarticularis above (upper small arrow). The inferior facet of L4 approximates the superior facet of SI (open arrows).

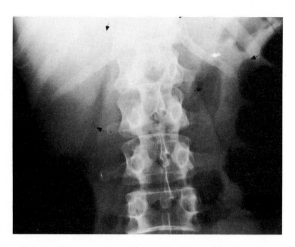

Fig. 2-32. Densities of the soft tissues may be misleading. The left kidney (solid arrows left upper abdomen) is identified, although partly obscured by gas in the colon and stomach. The outline of what might be mistakenly thought to be the right kidney is seen (solid arrows). However, this actually represents fat in the renal bed, the margin of the liver, and the edge of the gallbladder, all resting along the course of the psoas margins. The right kidney was removed 10 years before this film.

is a defect in a portion of the lamina. This allows the vertebral bodies to slip forward, one on top of the other.

The lower ribs and costal cartilages are well seen on films of the abdomen and should always be carefully studied. The irregular calcifications commonly seen in the costal cartilages may be mistaken for intra-abdominal calcifications. Frequent errors result from mistaking such calcifications for kidney stones or gallstones. For this reason, it is necessary to remember that the abdomen is a three-dimensional structure depicted in two dimensions. It is vital to think from "skin to skin" when studying the films. Amputation of the lateral portion of one of the twelfth ribs is a good clue that previous surgery has been performed on one or both kidneys. Since removal of the kidney may leave behind the fat that is normally around the kidney, it is possible to erroneously identify a kidney as present when it is, in fact, absent (Fig. 2-32). The only roentgenographic hint of such surgery may be the resection of the distal end of a twelfth rib.

The outlines of the muscles may provide a clue to abnormality. On the routine film of the abdomen, the iliopsoas margins contrasted against the retroperitoneal fat can usually be identified. Loss of the radiolucency of the fat from starvation, infiltration by tumor, or fluid will obscure the psoas margin. One should routinely attempt to identify the psoas margins when viewing an abdominal film. The fat layer between the abdominal musculature and the peritoneum (properitoneal fat line) is seen along the lateral aspect of the abdomen. Absence of this fat is most commonly the result of excess intra-abdominal fluid, or ascites, but it may result from starvation or edema.

The abdominal contents may be studied by changing the contrast within the

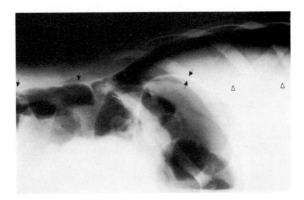

Fig. 2-33. Free air within the peritoneal cavity rises to the uppermost portion of the abdomen. With the patient lying in the decubitus position the radiolucency of gas collects above the liver with an air-fluid level (open arrows) crossing the liver. The stomach is distended with gas as well, and the thickness of the wall of the stomach is observed (opposing solid arrows). The outer margin of the colon (lower solid arrows) is also shown as the result of the gas being on the outside of the viscus. This occurrence is usually the result of a rupture of one of the hollow viscera in the abdomen.

abdomen by introducing gas. Intraperitoneal insufflation outlines the uterus and ovaries (gynecography). Following abdominal surgery, there is frequently some gas present in the abdomen after the incision has been closed. It is common, therefore, to see free air within the abdomen on roentgenograms taken shortly after abdominal surgery. Unless there has been an artificial introduction of gas into the peritoneal cavity or the patient is in the postoperative state, no free air should be present within the abdomen. If free gas is seen, it indicates the rupture of a hollow viscus, which may be the colon, stomach, or small bowel. This can be demonstrated roentgenographically by placing the patient in a position that will allow the gas to collect in one area. If the film is taken with the patient erect the gas collects beneath the leaves of the diaphragm and appears as a sharply defined radiolucent crescent. However, individuals who are extremely ill cannot be placed erect. If the patient is allowed to lie on one side, the gas will collect on the other side of the abdomen and can be demonstrated roentgenographically (Fig. 2-33). Occasionally free air within the abdominal cavity can be shown by having the patient lie on his back and then directing the beam horizontally. The gas is observed behind the anterior abdominal wall.

Hepatopancreatic system

The liver and pancreas are considered as a unit since the interaction between these organs is a frequent component of disease. The alteration from normal most frequently seen on films is increase in size. The liver is quite large and its position relative to other intraperitoneal structures makes it possible to determine its size directly. Increase in the size of the liver produces downward displacement of the hepatic flexure of the colon and may displace the stomach to the

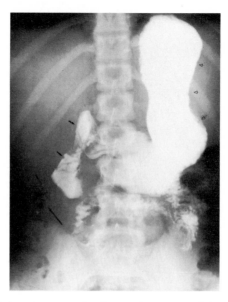

Fig. 2-34. Deformity of the viscera results from enlargement of intra-abdominal organs. The spleen (open arrows) and liver (short solid arrows) are both enlarged. The duodenal bulb and descending duodenum are displaced and deformed by the enlarged liver. The hepatic flexure of the colon (long solid arrow) is displaced downward by the liver. The margin of the stomach which rests against the spleen is also deformed by the splenic enlargement. The soft tissue margins of the liver and the spleen can be identified roentgenographically, but the localization and evaluation of size is more accurate when the intestinal tract is filled with barium. The deformities produced by extrinsic pressure may at times be difficult to distinguish from intrinsic disease of the intestinal tract.

left (Fig. 2-34). Common causes of liver enlargement are excess fluid and edema from infection, vascular stasis from cardiac failure, and infiltration of abnormal tissues by metastatic cancer or lymphoma. Pancreatic enlargement is demonstrable primarily by opacification of the adjoining structures; the usual method is the oral administration of an opaque substance which delineates the stomach and duodenum (Fig. 2-35).

Naturally occurring density changes may also indicate disease. In the liver, these changes usually consist of calcification within areas of healed infection, cysts, or metastatic tumor. The most common calcification in the region of the liver is calcified gallstones in the gallbladder. The pancreas often reflects abnormality by calcification, which is frequently a manifestation of chronic inflammation of the pancreas.

The intrinsic density of the ducts of the liver can be artificially altered (see Fig. 2-7). This alteration can be accomplished by several methods, the most common of which is intravenous cholangiography. An iodinated compound which is injected into the veins is selectively excreted by the liver. The ducts inside and outside the liver extending to the gallbladder and the intestinal tract become opacified. Severe liver dysfunction prevents ductal opacification because the

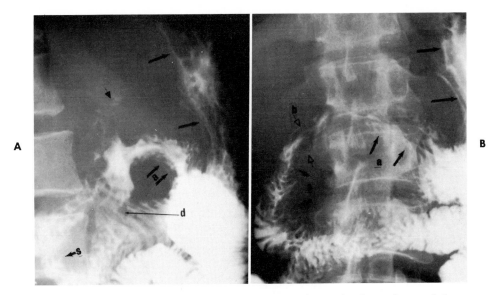

Fig. 2-35. Enlargement of the pancreas (in this instance the result of pseudocyst of the pancreas) may produce severe distortion of the adjoining structures. **A,** In the oblique projection of a G.I. series the posterior wall of the stomach (broad solid arrows) is displaced away from the spine. The gastric antrum (*a* between solid arrows) is elevated and impressed from the inferior aspect. The descending limb of the duodenum (duodenal sweep, *s*) is stretched, with the mucosa flattened. The horizontal limb of the duodenum (*d*) shows stretching of the mucosa pointing to the site of adhesion formation. The solid arrow behind the stomach points to calcific deposits in the pancreas indicative of chronic pancreatitis. **B,** In the P-A projection much of the same deformity is seen with the gastric antrum (*a* between arrows) being faintly identified and flattened. The body of the stomach (longer solid arrows) shows pressure along its medial aspect. The duodenal bulb (*b*, open arrows) lies to the right of the midline and is demonstrated by gas. This is somewhat deformed. The duodenal sweep (*s*) shows the same deformity seen in the oblique projection. Any mass lesion, such as lymph nodes or other tumors behind the stomach, can produce similar findings.

excretion is inadequate. Transhepatic cholangiography may then be used. A needle is inserted directly into the liver, and contrast medium is injected into the ducts. These methods opacify only the ductal systems and do not demonstrate the parenchyma of the liver. However, radioisotopes permit liver scanning and partial evaluation of the parenchyma of the liver. The pancreas is not as easily studied as the liver, although occasionally the pancreatic ducts may opacify. Work is in progress to derive techniques which will provide studies of the pancreas similar to those currently available for the liver.

Oral cholecystography is the most frequently used procedure for artificial density induction in the hepatopancreatic system. An iodinated compound is taken orally by the patient. It is excreted by the liver and concentrates within the gallbladder. The form of the gallbladder, the presence or absence of gallstones (Fig. 2-36), and some evaluation of the gallbladder's ability to concentrate bile are all studied. The gallbladder may also be opacified by intravenous cholangiography. This is a passive opacification and does not evaluate the gall-

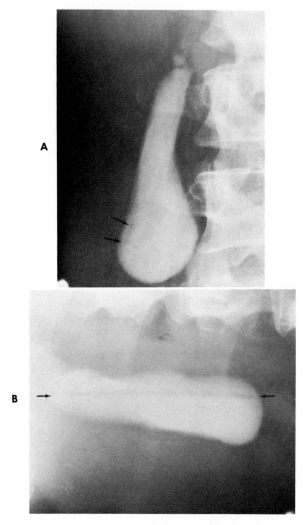

Fig. 2-36. A, Artificially increased density in the gallbladder (oral cholecystogram) shows multiple small lucencies (arrows) in the oblique prone projection. **B,** When the patient lies on the right side and a film is taken parallel to the floor the gallstones form a radiolucent line between the arrows. The bile lying below the gallstones is more concentrated and therefore has a greater specific gravity than the gallstones. The opacified bile that lies above the gall stones is less concentrated, therefore, less opaque.

bladder's ability to function. In oral cholecystography, the gallbladder is studied to determine its size, irregular filling, failure of filling, displacement, and appearance of the wall.

Inflammatory disease of either the pancreas or the liver may cause response in the adjoining tissues. Pleural effusion and abnormalities of the lungs may ensue.

Gastrointestinal system

Possible abnormalities of the gastrointestinal tract are the most frequent indications for routine films of the abdomen. The intestinal tract, however, is one of the most difficult intra-abdominal structures to study by plain roentgenographic methods. There is very little contrast between the structure of the bowel and the adjoining tissues unless the bowel contains gas or has been artificially opacified. Without changing the radiodensity, it is not possible to adequately study the intestinal tract.

Artificially induced radiodensity of the intestinal tract is the most common contrast study performed in roentgenology. The kind of examination chosen is adapted to help solve the problem. Thus, a study of the upper gastrointestinal system, commonly known as a G.I. series, is designed to evaluate the esophagus, stomach, duodenum, and proximal portion of jejunum. A small bowel series demonstrates the small bowel distal to the stomach by means of delayed films. A small bowel series should be used if there is a question of inflammation of the jejunum or the ileum. The barium enema and pneumocolon are designed to study the colon and the distal portion of the ileum after reflux occurs through the ileocecal valve. The barium enema is accomplished by using barium sulfate suspension as an enema fluid. If air is introduced through the rectum after the introduction of some barium sulfate suspension, a double contrast study of the colon (pneumocolon) is produced (see Fig. 2-7).

One of the basic points to remember is that in using barium sulfate in the intestinal tract, only the lumen of the viscus is being delineated. A column of barium or air or both is created, with the wall of the intestinal tract wrapped around the column. The outer wall of the viscus is not directly demonstrated. To show the outer wall of the viscus, techniques such as injecting air into the abdominal cavity or roentgenographic techniques utilizing high kilovoltage must be used. The thickness of the wall of the bowel can be judged in part by the distance separating the lumina of the adjoining loops of the bowel.

Characteristics studied

Some considerations of the gastrointestinal tract are:
1. Form. Is the structure smooth or irregular? Does the wall show retraction or protrusion from either adhesions or diverticula?
2. Consistency. Is the wall pliable or rigid, and is the viscus mobile or fixed?
3. Function. Is peristalsis present? How frequent are the peristaltic waves, and what is the depth of the waves?

Many of these factors can only be postulated on the basis of plainfilm studies,

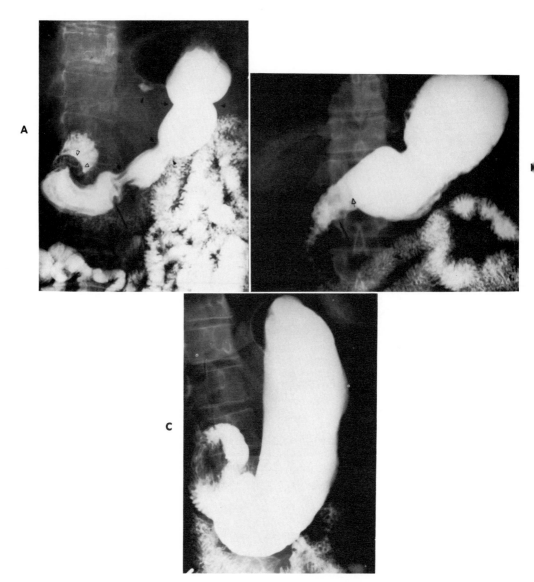

Fig. 2-37. A, Oblique projection of a gastrointestinal study with barium opacifying the stomach. While no acute disease is identified, there are several coincidental findings. Projecting inferiorly from the gas-filled fundus of the stomach is a small diverticulum (upper solid arrow). There are several peristaltic waves along the course of the stomach (opposing small solid arrows). Along the greater curvature of the antrum there is a deformity thought to be the result of adhesions (long arrow). Multiple films are needed to be sure that these findings are constant. Some prolapse of gastric mucosa into the duodenal bulb is present (open arrows). The mucosa of the duodenum, jejunum, and ileum appear normal. The thickness of the wall of the small bowel is that distance which separates the mucosa between adjoining loops. **B,** The antrum of the stomach and the region of the pyloric canal (open arrow) lie fairly high in the abdomen, compared to **A.** The duodenal bulb (long solid arrow) seems relatively small and points inferiorly. This is a normal variation (horizontal stomach). This is usually seen in individuals of rather robust habitus. **C,** The stomach is J shaped, with an upward pointing duodenal bulb. This is a normal variation and is of no significance.

A
B

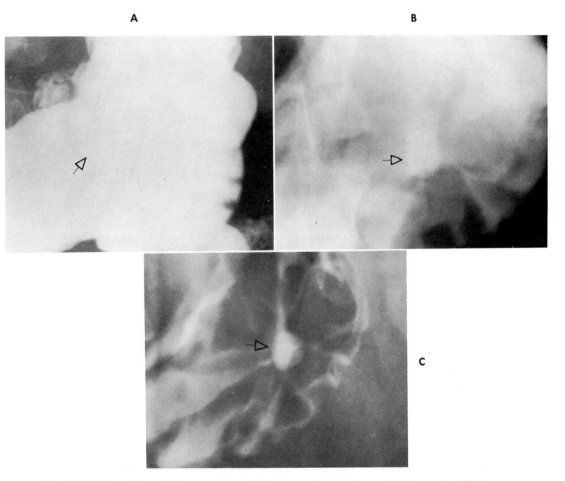

C

Fig. 2-38. Three films of the same area of the stomach are shown. **A,** On routine filming a vague collection of barium (open arrow) is seen to project through the stomach, representing an ulcer crater. **B,** With some pressure against the stomach the barium is partly displaced and the ulcer crater becomes more visible. **C,** If the patient is rotated so that the barium flows by gravity to other portions of the stomach and air rises to the region of the ulcer, its configuration and the changes in the adjoining area of the mucosa are much more easily seen. Such change in contrast is easily accomplished at the time of fluoroscopy. The appearance of the mucosal folds would indicate that this is a benign rather than a malignant ulcer.

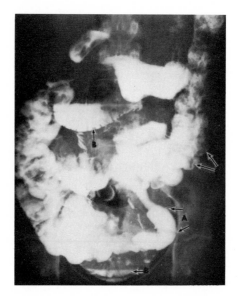

Fig. 2-39. Film of the small bowel. There are abnormal loops of poorly defined mucosa (*A*) and dilated loops of bowel with air fluid levels (*B*). The haustral pattern of the colon in the transverse portion appears rather saccular. These findings are characteristic of a collagen disease (scleroderma), and represent distortion both of form and function of the bowel.

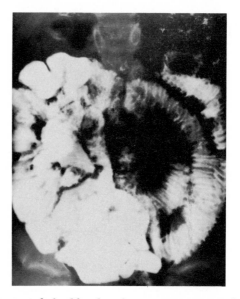

Fig. 2-40. The bowel is irregularly dilated with very coarse mucosal folds and thick walls. This appearance is expected in inflammatory disease and, in this patient, represents regional enteritis.

so that some form of dynamic roentgenography is needed for a complete study. Techniques available for the study include fluoroscopy, cineroentgenography, videotape recording, and pressure recording. If an abnormality is detected, an attempt should be made to determine whether it is intrinsic or extrinsic in origin.

The continuity of the column of barium outlining the lumen of the viscus may be interrupted. Such discontinuity may result from obstruction of the lumen or abnormal motility of the intestinal tract. Abnormal communications, such as fistulae or postoperative anastomoses, also produce discontinuity. Some variations are shown in Fig. 2-37.

The lining of the bowel is easily demonstrated, since the barium sulfate is in direct apposition to it. Small areas of loss of mucosa (ulcer) or excess tissues (tumor) can be seen. In order to fully demonstrate abnormalities, a profile view is required. Fig. 2-38 shows a gastric ulcer that would be hidden if it were not recorded tangentially or if the overlying barium were not displaced away from the ulcer crater. If the mucosa is infiltrated by tumor or edema, thickening and irregular walls will result. Inflammation or idiopathic mucosal thickening can produce the same findings (Figs. 2-39 and 2-40). On occasions, the mucosal lining becomes atrophic, and if the muscular wall is also thin, the folds of lining become less prominent. If only the mucosa is atrophic, the folds of the lining which result from the muscular coat are accentuated.

Excess mucosal lining presents as irregular polypoid masses that may result from edema or tumor and may be benign or malignant (Fig. 2-41).

The pneumocolon shows the lining of the colon very well. In the other portions of the bowel, this type of contrast is more difficult to induce artificially.

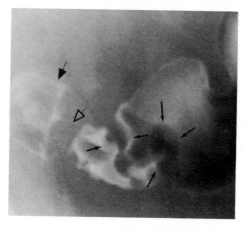

Fig. 2-41. Evaluation of the pattern of the mucosa of the stomach is accomplished by either barium or air and barium contrast. The polypoid thickening of the gastric mucosa in the distal portion of the stomach (small arrows) apparently results from inflammation. The pyloric channel (open arrow) lies just distal to the antrum and appears small since a peristaltic wave has just passed through this area. The duodenal bulb (solid arrow) is outlined by gas and barium enabling visualization of the mucosal lining.

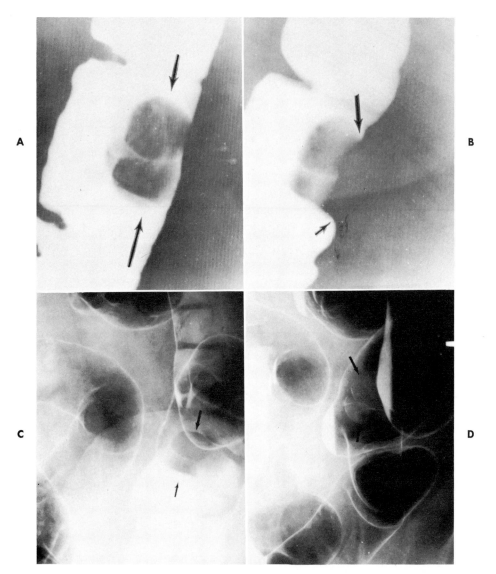

Fig. 2-42. The search for abnormal masses in the colon is accomplished by using both positive and negative contrast. **A,** The barium surrounds the polyp which becomes radiolucent in the central portion of the barium column (solid arrows). **B,** If the patient is rotated somewhat the attachment of the polyp to the bowel wall is seen; the solid arrows show the barium surrounding the base of the polyp. **C,** If air is introduced in addition, the polyp begins to appear as a soft tissue density superiorly (upper arrow) while still surrounded by barium inferiorly and is a negative density (lower arrow). **D,** When the barium has been replaced by air the polyp appears as a soft tissue density (solid arrows) and, therefore, more radiodense than the adjoining gas-filled bowel. This illustration demonstrates the value of pneumocolon and shows the relative change in density that may occur according to the surrounding substance. Change in density and change in form are both used in this instance.

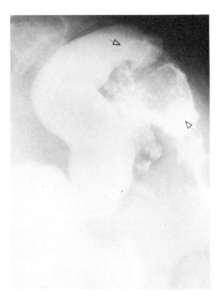

Fig. 2-43. A large lesion may be quite satisfactorily identified (open arrows). It represents a rather large polypoid tumor mass, in this instance, a villus adenoma which may become quite large.

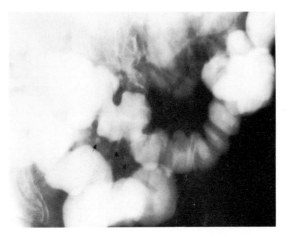

Fig. 2-44. Pockets of mucosa may project outward through the bowel wall and become filled with barium (diverticula, solid arrows). This condition represents change in form of the colonic wall. Such pockets usually are asymptomatic but may occasionally give rise to bleeding and partial obstruction.

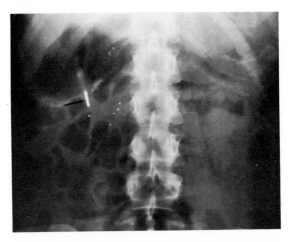

Fig. 2-45. Occasionally, accidental opacification of the intestinal tract results from ingestion of opaque material. A mercury thermometer was broken off in the mouth and the tip swallowed (solid arrow). The use of serial films will show the passage of such opaque material through the bowel.

The stomach normally contains some gas, so that by proper positioning of the patient, double contrast studies of portions of the stomach can be obtained. Figs. 2-42 and 2-43 show the comparative appearance of a polyp with and without the use of double contrast studies. Occasionally, it is easier to show the pattern of the lining of the bowel with less barium.

Alteration in the density of the barium sulfate results from dilution. Obstruction of the bowel, retained fluid from preparatory enemas, or ingestion of fluid as part of the examination may produce excess fluid in the intestinal tract, the usual cause of dilution. The examination is less satisfactory, since the dilution of the barium prevents good mucosal coating and may affect the motility and continuity of the barium column.

Knowledge of the usual position, and contour of the various parts of the intestinal tract becomes important (Fig. 2-44). Displacement of parts of the intestinal tract by masses within the abdomen is one of the commonly used methods of detecting an abnormality (see Fig. 2-35). Congenital malformation, retraction by adhesions, or excess intraperitoneal fluid may be manifested by altered position of the loops of the bowel.

Abnormal radiopacity of the intestinal tract may occur. Ingestion of foreign bodies such as lead shot or more bizarre objects can provide very entertaining roentgenograms (Fig. 2-45). Occasionally, medicinal substances such as bismuth or contrast medium from gallbladder studies may be present in the intestinal tract and may be shown on abdominal roentgenograms. Calcifications in the lumen or walls of the intestines are infrequent findings but may result from peritoneal abnormalities as in meconium ileus (along the walls) or gallstone ileus (in the lumen). Tumors of the stomach and rectum occasionally calcify (Fig. 2-46),

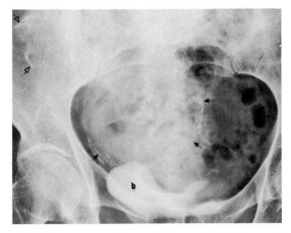

Fig. 2-46. Unusual calcifications show as roentgenographic densities. In this patient, there are two such calcific deposits. The larger one (solid arrows) represents a mucocele of the appendix, while the open arrows show calcifications in a tumor of the cecum. The bladder is opacified (*b*) as the result of an intravenous urogram and shows deformity from the adjoining tumor mass.

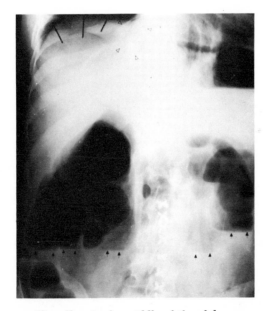

Fig. 2-47. This is a story-telling film. In the middle of the abdomen are metallic crosses that represent postsurgical skin clips. When these are present the patient has undergone recent surgery. The long arrows in the upper portion of the picture point to gas beneath the diaphragmatic leaf, another result of recent surgery on the abdomen. Just medial to this (open arrows) is a density that represents atelectasis of the right lower lobe of the lung. Multiple fluid levels within the intestinal tract (small solid arrows) indicate a bowel obstruction. The patient is erect. The total abnormalities, therefore, represent postoperative bowel obstruction, free intraperitoneal air, and atelectasis of the right lower lobe. Changes in location and density are the roentgenographic clues.

A   B

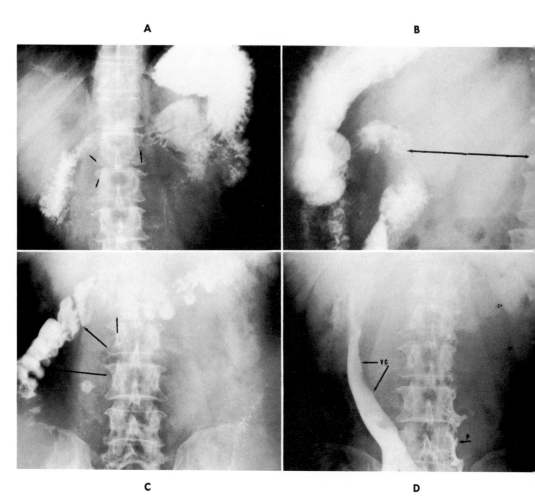

C   D

Fig. 2-48. A retrogastric, retroperitoneal mass can be identified by distortion of the intestinal tract. **A,** The stomach is elevated, the duodenal bulb is pushed up and to the right, and the horizontal limb of the duodenum is flattened (short arrows). **B,** In the lateral projection displacement anteriorly by the retrogastric mass (solid arrow), indicates the retrogastric location. **C,** The mass is sufficiently large to cause impression on the inferior medial aspect of the hepatic flexure (arrows). **D,** In addition, the artificially opacified vena cava (*VC*) is displaced to the right. The open arrows show the margin of the mass projecting to the left and impressing the inferior margin of the kidney, partially outlined by excretion of the iodinated compound. The paraspinal plexus (*P*) is opacified, showing the partial obstruction of the inferior vena cava by the large tumor.

but phleboliths (calcification in the veins) or calcified lymph nodes are more frequent findings.

The wall of the intestinal tract may sometimes be abnormally radiolucent, resulting from the penetration of the bowel wall by gas (pneumatosis cystoides intestinalis). The margins of the intestine may appear increased in density if extravasation of the contrast medium through a perforated wall occurs or if gas is present in the abdomen.

Roentgenographic examinations of the intestinal tract should include a preliminary plain film of the abdomen (Fig. 2-47). This film provides a base line for comparison with the additional films taken during a more definitive study.

Identifying the various structures demonstrated on a gastrointestinal series or a barium enema is easier if the film sequence is studied as if fluoroscopy were being performed. Thus, the sequence should be viewed in the following order: the esophagus, cardia of the stomach, pars media of the stomach, antrum of the stomach, duodenal bulb, descending limb of the duodenum, and the proximal small bowel.

The contour of the bowel lumen, the continuity of barium meal, and the distance between the filled lumen of adjoining loops of the small bowel are indications of wall thickness, pliability and functional ability. Some indirect evidence of bowel function can thereby be obtained. Perigastric masses may increase the distance between the stomach and the transverse colon. If the bowel wall is infiltrated, the function will be impaired (see Fig. 2-39). In viewing the films of a barium enema, the rectum, rectosigmoid, sigmoid, descending colon, transverse colon, and ascending colon should be studied in that order. This sequence represents the order of demonstration at the time of fluoroscopy. The splenic flexure, hepatic flexure, and ileocecal valve require special attention if an examination is to be complete. There are focal areas in which the colon angles and may be somewhat narrowed. These areas occur when the position of the colon changes from intraperitoneal to retroperitoneal. The transverse mesocolon and the sigmoid mesocolon result from the intraperitoneal position of the segments of the colon.

The postevacuation film shows the mucosal pattern of the colon most effectively. Also, persistence of "filling" defects in the lumen of the colon seen on postevacuation films, as well as films in which the colon is filled with barium, helps differentiate between tumors and other intraluminal material.

The gastrointestinal tract lies against many intra-abdominal structures and the abdominal wall. This system serves as an indicator of soft tissue abnormalities in the adjoining structures. Thus, a gastrointestinal series and small bowel study, or barium enema, may assist in evaluating growth or regression of tumor masses extrinsic to the bowel or enlargement of other intra-abdominal organs (Fig. 2-48).

Lymphatic system and spleen

Intra-abdominal lymph nodes are usually invisible on routine roentgenograms unless there is an alteration of their normal structure. For instance, a change in

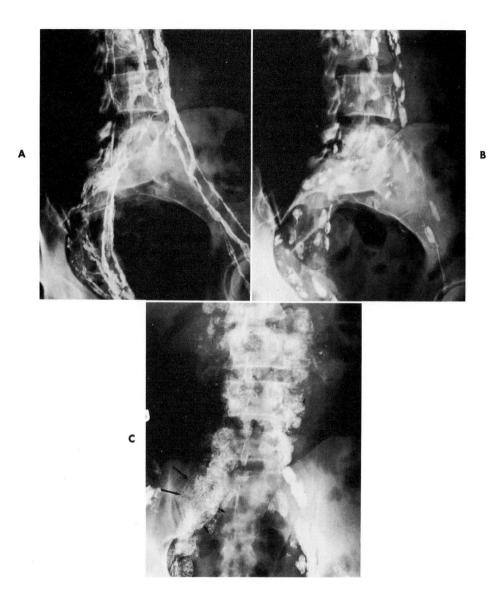

Fig. 2-49. If an iodinated oily compound is injected into the interdigital lymphatics of the foot the lymphatic channels (**A**) and the retroperitoneal lymph nodes (**B**) become opacified. Tumor obstruction or involvement of the nodes can thereby be detected. These lymphatic channels and the lymph nodes are considered normal. **C**, In contrast to the appearance of the nodes in **B**, the lymph nodes (solid arrows) are enlarged and irregular. This appearance is indicative of lymphoma, in this instance, Hodgkins' disease.

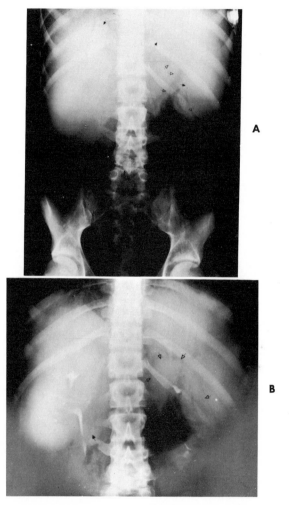

Fig. 2-50. A, With enlargement of the liver and spleen the gas bubble of the stomach may be displaced downward (open arrows). The margins of the liver and spleen can be identified (solid arrows). The twelfth rib on the right was resected at the time of drainage of a sub-phrenic abscess. The body of the fourth lumbar vertebra is destroyed by inflammatory disease. **B,** The left kidney is displaced downward as compared to the right kidney (open arrows). On the right the density at the tip of the solid arrow represents calculi within the gallbladder. On a single film, therefore, abnormality of the osseous system, urinary system, and hepatopan-creatic splenic system are all identified.

density, usually calcific, may result from a previous infection. Nodes that are altered in this manner have a rather characteristic "popcorn" appearance. If certain contrast media are injected into the lymphatics between the toes (lymphangiography), the media will traverse the lymph channels and collect in the lymph nodes, thus rendering the nodes opaque. Normal and abnormal lymphangiograms are illustrated in Fig. 2-49.

If the lymph nodes are enlarged, they may appear as a soft tissue mass with their density contrasted against the retroperitoneal fat. Displacement of adjoining structures, such as kidneys, ureters, bladder, or sections of the gastrointestinal tract also allows detection of enlarged nodes. The contour of intra-abdominal lymph node masses is difficult to assess without lymphangiography, but lobulation may occasionally be identifiable on a routine roentgenogram.

As part of the hematopoietic-lymphatic system, the spleen may reflect an important diagnostic clue in cases of abnormality of the lymphatic system, for example, leukemia. The size, contour, and margination of the spleen should be studied on any film of the abdomen. Parasplenic inflammatory disease will blur the margins of the spleen and, in addition, will frequently affect the adjoining structures such as the stomach (Fig. 2-50). As with the other intra-abdominal structures, the spleen and lymph nodes may be displaced by abnormal adjoining tissues such as pancreatic masses and tumors. It is possible to have accessory spleens, and in this case the abnormal density can be mistaken for lymph nodes or other abnormal tissue. Tumors or infection represent common disease processes of the lymphatic-splenic system.

Genitourinary system

Normally, all of the structures of the urinary system have the density of soft tissue. Contrast to the surrounding radiolucent fat or artificially induced contrast is required to show individual organs. (The fat in the retroperitoneal space and renal beds makes possible the demonstration of the nonopacified renal structures on the plain films of the abdomen.) Calculi, nephrocalcinosis, postinflammatory calcification, and tumorous calcification are all naturally occurring variations in density and permit identification of certain areas of the structures (Fig. 2-51). Occasionally, abnormal or excessive fat deposits occur, thereby producing an unusual radiolucency.

Whether the margins of the kidneys are sharply defined or not is of importance in study of the kidneys. Lack of such definition may result from either the loss of retroperitoneal fat from malnutrition or edema in the fat reducing the sharp contrast of the kidney parenchyma (Fig. 2-52). This is assessable on the plain film studies but can be enhanced by retroperitoneal pneumography which produces increased contrast around the margins of the kidney. This technique also makes possible the study of the size, contour, and margination of the adrenals. Sharpness of the psoas margins and bladder margins also can be studied.

Artificial contrast is commonly introduced for the opacification of the urinary tract. Although many techniques can be used, intravenous urography is the most

A

B

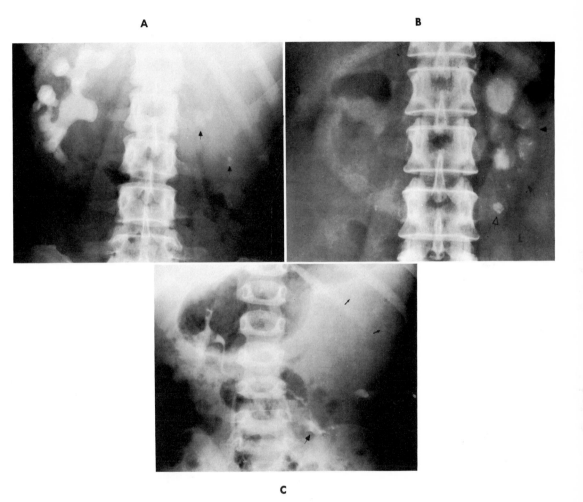

C

Fig. 2-51. A, A spectacular density change may occur within the kidneys. The right kidney shows delineation of the collecting structures by extensive calcification (staghorn calculus). Smaller calcific deposits are present in the kidney on the opposite side (small arrows). **B,** The plain film of the abdomen shows irregular densities collected in the region of the left kidney (solid arrows) and irregular calcifications lying below the kidney (open arrow). Another irregular calcification is observed on the right side (open arrow). The changes in the left kidney result from severe inflammatory destruction of the kidney (putty kidney); calcifications in the lymph nodes and a calcific deposit in the right upper quadrant, representing a gallstone, are incidental findings. The left kidney is observed to be changed in both size and density. **C,** A large mass in the left upper quadrant of the abdomen displaces the collecting structures of the left kidney (low solid arrow). It contains faint calcific deposits (small solid arrows). This is calcification within a large Wilms' tumor of the left kidney.

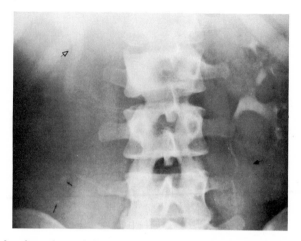

Fig. 2-52. There has been loss of the roentgenographic margin of the right psoas muscle as compared to the left (solid arrows), and faint deposits of calcium are seen in the right flank (small arrows). The right ureter is broad, and there is some dilatation of the renal pelvis (open arrow). These are the signs of a retroperitoneal perinephric abscess. The associated increased density of the body of the second lumbar vertebra is probably coincidental; it could result from a previously healed infection.

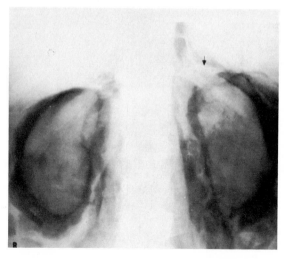

Fig. 2-53. Gas introduced into the retroperitoneal tissues through the presacral space will dissect upward and outline the kidneys. The adrenals (solid arrow) can be identified as soft tissue masses superimposed upon the upper pole of the kidney. The gas in this case is partly trapped in Gerota's fascia and will not ascend into the adrenal area as completely as usual. This is an example of artificially reduced density.

frequent. An iodinated organic compound is injected into the vein, the material passes through the arterial circulation of the kidney and is filtered out of the bloodstream. The collecting systems that are part of the renal parenchyma as well as the bladder become radiodense as the urine containing the opaque medium is excreted. Early in the phase of excretion, the contrast medium within the kidney parenchyma produces an increase in the kidney density. This is called a nephrogram. Lack of opacification of a certain area of the kidney or prolonged opacification of the kidney indicates an abnormality (Figs. 2-53 to 2-55). Some evaluation of the renal function is possible by intravenous urography since the kidney must be able to excrete and concentrate the medium. Prolonged increased density and the delayed onset of excretion of the contrast medium are indicative of poor function. Retrograde pyelography, and cystography opacify the drainage pathways by the placement of catheters into the ureters by way of the bladder and the injection of contrast medium (Figs. 2-56 and 2-57). A needle may be inserted into an area of the kidney that may contain a cyst. Direct injection of contrast medium then shows the character of the cyst and its wall (Fig. 2-58). Intravenous urography demonstrates the lining of the hollow viscus and opacifies, in the following order, the fornices, the calyces, infundibula, renal pelvis, ureter, bladder, and urethra.

The major criteria for judging normality of the urinary tract are the rate and degree of excretion and the configuration of the opacified viscera. Distortion of the artificially opacified urinary drainage system may result from an intrinsic disease of the system, such as congenital abnormalities, tumors, infection, spasm, or obstruction. The retroperitoneal position of the urinary tract provides an excellent opportunity for the demonstration of abnormalities of the soft tissues of

Text continued on p. 131.

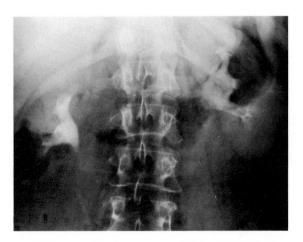

Fig. 2-54. At the end of 5 minutes after the start of an intravenous urogram it can be seen that the right kidney is appreciably denser than the left. Such differential excretion can be the result of infection, decreased blood flow as from arteriosclerosis, or obstruction of the ureter. It is the variation in density between the right and left kidneys that indicates that the left is abnormal.

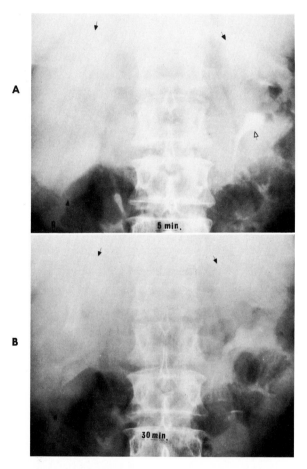

Fig. 2-55. Persistent opacification of the kidneys may occur as the result of obstruction. **A,** Five minutes after the start of an intravenous urogram, the right kidney is appreciably denser than the left (solid arrows indicate upper and lower poles of kidneys). The left renal pelvis (open arrow) is identified. **B,** At the end of 30 minutes there continues to be an increased density in the right kidney compared to the left. Some excretion of the contrast medium into the collecting system is noted. The prolonged opacification of the right kidney results from an acute obstruction of the right ureter by a calculus.

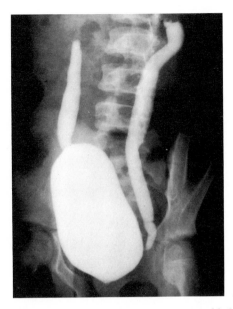

Fig. 2-56. Direct injection of opaque material into the urinary bladder (cystogram) shows the distensibility and contour of the urinary bladder. If there is lack of sphincteric competence at the junction of the ureters and the bladder, reflux into the ureters may occur as is observed here.

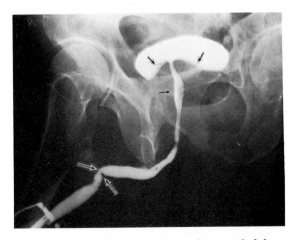

Fig. 2-57. The lower portion of the urinary tract may be opacified by injection of contrast medium through the urethra into the bladder. The male urethra is well shown. There is impression on the base of the bladder (small arrows) by an enlarged prostate. The large arrow points to the region of the prostatic urethra. In the midurethral area apposing arrows point to the site of urethral stricture as the result of previous infection. The change in form of the urethra enables evaluation of the adjoining tissues as well as the intrinsic structure of the urethra.

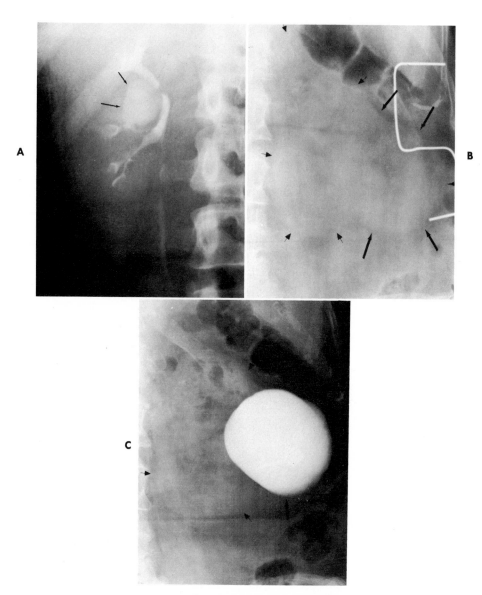

Fig. 2-58. A, Deformity of the collecting structures of the kidney is a diagnostic finding. In this instance, there is excess collection of the contrast medium in an area of cyst formation in the margin of the renal pelvis (peripelvic cyst, arrows). The collection of contrast medium indicates that this does, however, communicate with the renal pelvis. **B,** On the plain film of the abdomen the outline of the kidney (short arrows) is barely identifiable. Projecting laterally from the kidney (long arrows) is a smoothly defined rounded mass. A metallic marker has been placed on the skin to localize this area for introduction of a needle. **C,** Following the placement of a needle and the injection of an iodinated compound the renal outline is again seen (short arrows). The soft tissue mass is now opacified (long arrow) and represents a benign renal cyst.

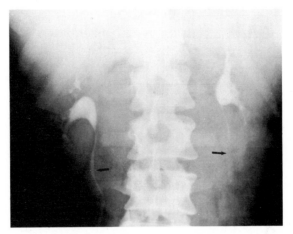

Fig. 2-59. Retroperitoneal masses can be demonstrated by opacification of the ureters, in this instance, by intravenous urography. The ureters are displaced laterally (arrows) by the midline lymph node enlargement from Hodgkins' disease.

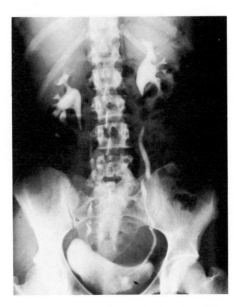

Fig. 2-60. An intravenous urogram shows a change in the size of the collecting structures and deformity of the bladder by an overlying soft tissue mass (open arrows). This represents an enlarged postpartum uterus. The opacified urine is entering the bladder through the uretero-vesical junction on the left (solid arrow) producing a waterfall effect. The densities in the right side of the abdomen are medicinal tablets in the course of the intestinal tract. The change in form and size is a normal physiologic alteration following pregnancy.

A   B

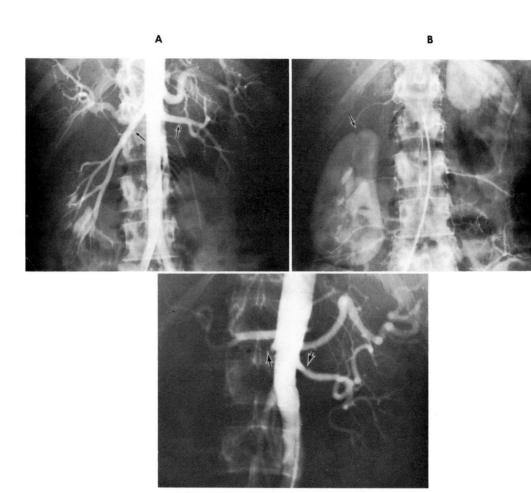

C

Fig. 2-61. **A,** Opacification of the renal arteries (arrows) is accomplished by means of an intra-aortic injection of an iodinated compound through a catheter. These renal arteries are normal. **B,** Shortly after injection, the parenchyma of the kidneys opacifies. The upper pole of the right kidney shows a small irregularity, probably as the result of persistent fetal lobulation (arrow). **C,** Disturbance of the renal arteries may produce either obstruction or irregularity. The right renal artery (solid arrow) fails to opacify because of fibromuscular hypertrophy (a thickening of the wall of the arteries). The left renal artery is less severely involved (open arrow). High blood pressure may be a complication.

the retroperitoneal space. Enlargement of the lymph nodes, retroperitoneal tumors, and infectious masses can be indirectly demonstrated by means of intravenous urograms (Fig. 2-59). Distortion or dilatation of the collecting systems, including the bladder, may be clues to the primary disease of the urinary tract or abnormalities in the adjoining tissues. The bladder normally shows some distortion in the female which is caused by the pressure of the uterus (Fig. 2-60). In the male, elevation of the floor of the bladder occurs with prostatic enlargement. Other causes of extrinsic pressure would be masses, distention of adjoining bowel by fluid, lymph nodes, or postoperative adhesion formation.

The size of the structures of the urinary system is important in the evaluation of normality. If one kidney is removed, the opposite kidney becomes enlarged as a result of the increased work placed upon it (compensatory hypertrophy). Edema or infiltration by abnormal tissue may cause increased size of the kidneys. Information is available giving the predicted size for the kidneys, but generally there is less than 1 cm. difference in the longitudinal axis of the right and left kidneys. Greater differences in the size of the kidneys warrant further study. Obstruction in the region of the ureters and bladder may cause dilatation of the more proximal portions of the collecting system. Lack of peristaltic action and loss of muscle tone are less common causes of distention of the ureters.

Decrease in the size of the kidneys frequently results from infection or decreased blood. The renal parenchyma becomes atrophic and scarred. The bladder may also be small or scarred as a result of infection. A postradiation effect will cause the same abnormality. Newer methods of study, including voiding cystourethrography, cineroentgenography, and arteriography allow evaluation of the function, size, and configuration of these various structures (Fig. 2-61).

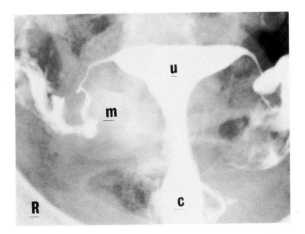

Fig. 2-62. Direct injection of an iodinated compound into the uterus (hysterosalpingography) passes through the cervix (*c*) to outline the uterine cavity (*u*). Extending laterally from the uterine cavity, the fallopian tubes surround the areas of the ovaries. Some of the contrast medium (*m*) has leaked into the right side of the pelvic peritoneal cavity to indicate that the tube is at least partially patent.

The genital tract should be viewed while assessing the urinary tract. The size of the uterus and ovaries is reflected in the bladder form. A more definitive evaluation of size, however, is accomplished by inducing an artificial radiolucency with intraperitoneal gas (pelvic pneumography or gynecography). Positive contrast medium may be injected directly into the uterine cavity by way of the vagina (hysterosalpingography) (Fig. 2-62). The contrast material passes through the fallopian tubes and eventually escapes into the intraperitoneal space. Therefore, the size and configuration of the gonadal structures can be accurately ascertained. Uterine enlargement is most frequently the result of pregnancy, but may also be caused by a benign tumor (Fig. 2-63). The contour of the uterus is helpful in determining the cause of enlargement. Lobulation indicates a tumor. The density of the uterus may change naturally to indicate disease. Ovarian enlargement usually reflects a cyst or tumor. Gynecography is required for adequate study of ovarian hypoplasia or infantile uteri which can result from hormonal imbalance (Figs. 2-64 to 2-66).

The size and configuration of the prostate produce an effect on the adjoining structures, primarily the bladder and urethra. Displacement, dilatation, or decreased size of these structures may be caused by abnormalities of the prostate. Knowing the characteristic location of prostatic calcifications, which are quite frequent, assists in differentiating them from bladder stones (Fig. 2-67).

The seminal vesicles normally are not identifiable unless previous infection

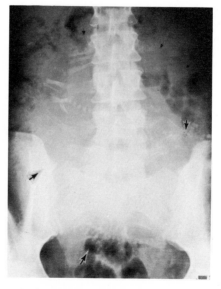

Fig. 2-63. The uterus is markedly enlarged (solid arrows). Lying within the uterine cavity are two fetal skeletons (open arrows). This represents twin pregnancies. The fetuses are in the transverse position; that is, the spines are parallel to the bottom of the film. The calcific density of the fetal skeleton is usually first detectable at approximately the fourth month of gestation. The present illustration is of approximately a sixth month stage.

has caused calcification of these structures. Vesiculography can be performed but is an infrequent examination since its general application and purpose remain somewhat in doubt.

Since the kidneys, uterus, and ovaries are solid organs, with the exception of the renal pelvis, irregularity of outline implies abnormal soft tissue, either a tumor or scar tissue. One exception to this is the left kidney, the so-called "dromedary kidney, which normally has a prominence on its lateral margin (Fig. 2-68). The pressure of the spleen against the superior lateral aspect of the left kidney causes this prominence. Smooth enlargement of the kidneys is more likely caused by edema, compensatory hypertrophy, or infiltration of abnormal tissue rather than primary neoplasm. Bladder wall irregularity may be caused by a diverticulum or by the effect of extrinsic pressure (Fig. 2-69). Irregular ureters frequently represent pressure by the adjacent soft tissues. Examples of this are retroperitoneal tumors, periureteral varices, enlarged lymph nodes, and so on. The ureters may occasionally have an irregular form because of an intrinsic disease such as scarring or tumor formation (Fig. 2-70).

Awareness of the normal location of the kidneys and bladder permits the assessment of the retroperitoneal structures. Normally, the left kidney lies higher than the right. The lower poles are anterior to the superior portion of the kidneys paralleling the psoas margins. The location of the kidneys is determined by the attitude of the body—in the erect position, the kidneys normally drop; however, if this does not occur, fixation from fibrosis or other diseases may be suspected.

Accessory kidneys occasionally occur, but the abnormal location of kidney tissues is usually caused by the failure of ascent of the kidneys. Ectopic location (pelvic kidney) and crossed ectopia, for instance, with the right kidney lying on the left side of the abdomen, are fairly common abnormalities (Fig. 2-71). The two kidneys may be fused, usually at their lower pole, producing a horseshoe

Text continued on p. 138.

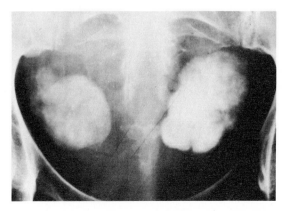

Fig. 2-64. Tumors within the genitourinary tract may become densely opaque as the result of dystrophic calcification. These bilateral ovarian cancers show extensive lobulated calcification.

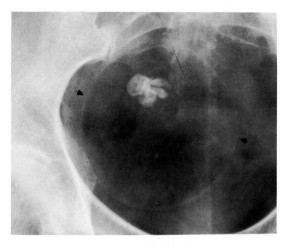

Fig. 2-65. Tumors are occasionally of mixed density. A fine rim of radiodensity (arrows) surrounds a ball of radiolucency within which lie irregular areas of calcification. This is a dermoid cyst of the ovary with radiolucency resulting from the excess fat. The irregular radiodensities therein are abortive teeth. The density of the tooth structure exceeds that of the adjoining osseous structure of the bony pelvis.

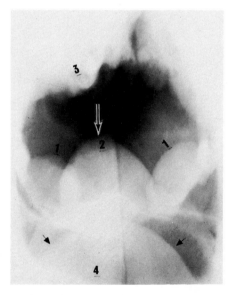

Fig. 2-66. By introduction of gas (nitrous oxide) into the peritoneal cavity, the soft tissue densities of the abdominal viscera can be made to contrast against the radiolucency of the gas. In the female pelvis, the uterus (*2*) is seen projecting above the urinary bladder (*4*) (short arrows). The ovaries are seen on either side (*1*) and the sigmoid colon is reflected posteriorly (*3*). The uterus shows minor lobulation (solid arrow) which represents a minor fibrous tumor in the wall of the uterus. The anatomic orientation is that looking down into the true pelvic space with the sacrum at the top of the film. Except for the minor uterine irregularity the study is considered normal.

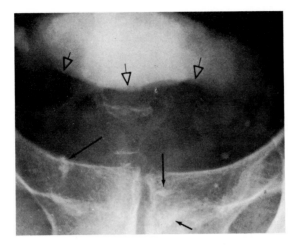

Fig. 2-67. Combined artificial and naturally occurring densities may assist in defining abnormalities. The prostate contains multiple areas of calcification (long solid arrows). In addition, the bladder, which is opacified as the result of intravenous urography, is elevated (open arrows) showing enlargement of the prostate. Calcifications in the prostate are quite common in older males.

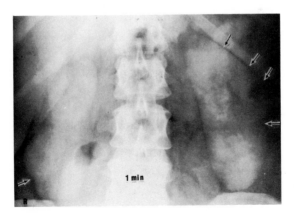

Fig. 2-68. The form of the kidneys is not always smooth. The left kidney, opacified 1 minute after the injection of iodinated compound into the vein, shows a rather prominent rounded margin (solid arrows). This represents developmental shaping from apposition to the spleen and is considered a dromedary kidney. The right kidney shows some irregularity in its lower pole (open arrow) which is scarring from previous infection.

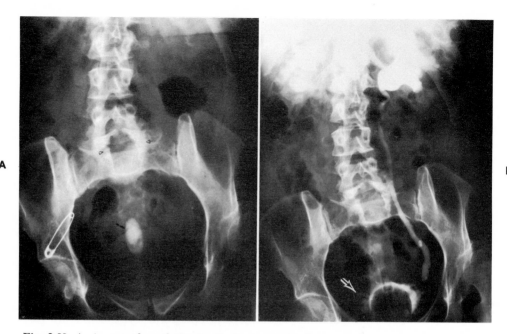

A

Fig. 2-69. A, An irregular calcific density is present in the true pelvic space (solid arrow). This represents a bladder calculus. The absence of the neural arches of the fifth lumbar and first and second sacral vertebrae (open arrow) indicates a meningomyelocele. A neurologic deficit has resulted with partial dislocation of the left hip. **B,** An intravenous urogram done on an earlier day shows irregularity of the bladder (diverticula) in which the calculus subsequently formed. The bladder is not opacified in the central portion because of the balloon of a retention catheter.

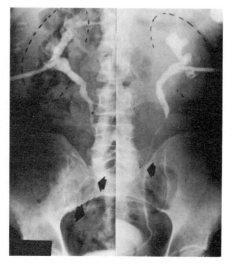

Fig. 2-70. Periureteral fibrosis may cause obstruction in the lower urinary tract, requiring tubes to be placed into the renal pelvis through the skin (nephrostomy). Retroperitoneal fibrosis has caused narrowing of the ureters (arrows).

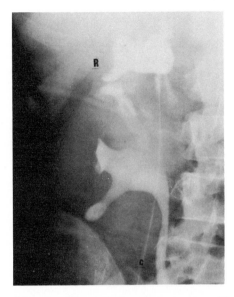

Fig. 2-71. Congenital mal-location of renal tissues may occur. The right kidney (*R*) is represented as a small superiorly placed renal structure. The larger kidney below represents the structure of the left kidney (*L*), which is totally placed on the right. The catheter (*c*) extends along the course of the right ureter. This represents an ectopic kidney with crossed fusion to the lower pole of the right kidney.

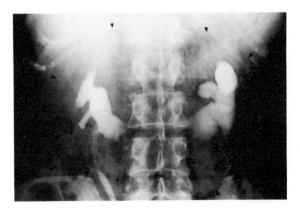

Fig. 2-72. A fairly common anomaly is fusion of the lower poles of the kidney (horseshoe kidney). The upper poles are outlined by the solid arrows. The crossed fusion mass is outlined by the lower solid arrows. The renal pelves (open arrow) point laterally.

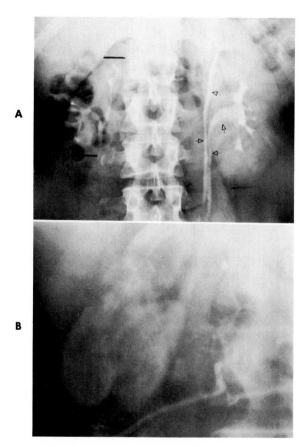

Fig. 2-73. A, The size of the kidneys may be sharply reduced as the result of infection. The longitudinal diameter of the right kidney (between the solid lines) is appreciably smaller than the left kidney, which has undergone some compensatory hypertrophy. The distance between the opacified calyces and renal cortex on the right compared to the left shows the loss of parenchyma on the right. In addition, there is major duplication of the drainage system on the left (open arrows). **B,** A renal arteriogram done on the same patient shows on the delayed phase the severity of the scarring of the right kidney with marked notch formation on the lower pole (arrow) and generally irregular opacity.

kidney (Fig. 2-72). A lateral rotation of the renal pelvis ensues and is easily identifiable on intravenous urograms.

One of the kidneys, an ovary, or the uterus may be congenitally absent or removed surgically. The duplication of the urinary drainage pathway is one of the more common anomalies of the mesenchymal tissues of the body. The degree of duplication varies from complete drainage pathway and renal parenchyma to partial duplication of the intrarenal drainage (Fig. 2-73).

REQUIRED READINGS

Squire, L. F.: Fundamentals of roentgenology, Cambridge, Mass., 1964, Harvard University Press.

Storch, C. B.: Fundamental aids in roentgen diagnosis, New York, 1951, Grune & Stratton, Inc.

Templeton, F. E.: X-ray examination of the stomach, Chicago, 1944, University of Chicago Press.

RECOMMENDED READINGS

Braasch, W. F., and Emmett, J. L.: Clinical urography, Philadelphia, 1951, W. B. Saunders Co.

Caffey, J.: Pediatric x-ray diagnosis, Chicago, 1961, Year Book Medical Publishers, Inc., pp. 499-646, 649-744.

Paul, L. W., and Juhl, J. H.: The essentials of roentgen interpretation, New York, 1964, Hoeber Medical Division, Harper & Row, Publishers, pp. 301-472, 475-529.

ADDITIONAL READING

Margulis, A. R.: Alimentary tract roentgenology, St. Louis, 1967, The C. V. Mosby Co.

3

APPENDICULAR AREAS

Summary of basic concepts

Diagnostic roentgenology of the appendicular areas involves three general categories of anatomic structures: soft tissues, articulations, and bones. The skeletal system is an indicator of the systemic and metabolic status of the body as a whole or locally and records previous systemic stress.

I. Soft tissue
   A. Components
      1. Skin
      2. Fat
      3. Muscle
      4. Fascia
      5. Ligaments and tendons
      6. Lymphatics
      7. Blood vessels
   B. Density
      1. Naturally occurring radiolucent (fat) against water density (muscle, ligaments, etc.)
         a. Subcutaneous fat and between muscle bundles
         b. Alterations of density
            (1) Increased radiolucency
               (a) Excess fat
               (b) Loss of muscle mass
            (2) Decreased radiolucency
               (a) Inanition
               (b) Fat necrosis
               (c) Edema
      2. Naturally occurring abnormality
         a. Calcific deposits
            (1) Blood vessels
               (a) Arteries: arteriosclerosis or systemic disease
               (b) Veins: phleboliths, varicosities, angiomas
            (2) Subcutaneous: dermatomyositis, scar
            (3) Ectopic bone formation following burns or varicose veins
         b. Soft tissue deposits: density of fat distorted (e.g., fibroma)
      3. Artificially increased
         a. Arteriography, venography, or lymphangiography

        b. Injection of contrast material into abnormal space as sinus tract

  C. Size

     1. Increased

         a. Dilated vessels

         b. Muscular hypertrophy

         c. Hematoma or tumor

         d. Overgrowth of soft tissue (e.g., heel pad in acromegaly)

     2. Decreased

         a. Atrophy

         b. Surgical removal

         c. Congenital absence

  D. Contour—abnormal

     1. Tumors—distortion adjoining tissues

     2. Rupture of tendons—"bunching" of muscles

     3. Vessels—dilatation or tortuosity with aging or disease

     4. Skin—reflects adjoining pressure, overgrowth, or edema

  E. Location and number

     1. Soft tissue planes or vessels displaced by adjoining masses

     2. Number of vessels identifiable

         a. Increased in tumors, malformations, collateral circulation from obstruction

         b. Decreased in occlusion

  F. Sharpness of definition

     1. Decreased: edema, inflammation, tumor

     2. Increased: excess fat

II. Articulations

  A. Components

     1. Cartilage

     2. Capsule

     3. Synovia

     4. Ligaments

     5. Fluid

  B. Density

     1. Naturally occurring (soft tissue)

         a. Contrast against increased density of bone

         b. Contrast against decreased density of fat

     2. Naturally occurring abnormality

         a. Calcification: hemorrhage, tumor, degeneration, metabolic disturbance —increased

         b. Vacuum phenomenon—decreased

     3. Artificially changed (arthrography)

         a. Increased: contrast medium injection

         b. Decreased: injection of gas

         c. Demonstrates joint cavity

  C. Size (width) of joint space

     1. Increased

         a. Dislocation—loss of support

        b. Effusion—increased pressure

        c. Acromegaly—increased cartilage

     2. Decreased (reduced cartilaginous thickness)

        a. Degeneration

        b. Postinflammatory change

        c. Posttraumatic change

  D. Contour and location

     1. Irregular articular cartilage

        a. Degeneration

        b. Postinflammatory change

        c. Posttraumatic change

     2. Bursa with excess fluid (effusion) displaces adjoining fat

  E. Loss of distinctness of margination

     1. Periarticular inflammatory disease with bone resorption

     2. Obliteration by edema

III. Skeletal system

  A. Components

     1. Epiphysis

     2. Epiphyseal ossification centers

     3. Metaphysis

     4. Diaphysis

     5. Cortex

     6. Medullary cavity

     7. Articulating surfaces

     8. Periosteum

     9. Endosteum

  B. Density

     1. Naturally occurring

        a. Radiodensity (whiteness) from calcium content

        b. Densest in cortex, but also dense in trabeculae of medullary cavity

        c. Increased by excess calcium deposit

     2. Naturally occurring abnormality

        a. Decreased density—reduced calcium content (most frequent abnormality)

        b. Increased density

           (1) Reactive hyperostosis

           (2) Chemical insult

           (3) Traumatic or inflammatory repair

           (4) Metastasis

           (5) Transverse lines of increased density (growth lines)—disturbed maturation while bone was forming

        c. Assessment

           (1) Extent: all bones, all of one bone, part of one bone, or part of several bones

           (2) Location: acute processes affect most metabolically active portion of bone (metaphysis)

           (3) Focal versus diffuse: systemic versus local disease

C. Size
  1. Reflects body size and hormonal influence
  2. Production
      a. Appositional bone deposit—periosteum: width
      b. Epiphyseal growth: length
      c. Enchondral—preformed in cartilage
      d. Apophyseal—ligamentous attachments: final form
  3. Abnormalities
      a. Epiphyseal disturbance: abnormal length and width
      b. Excess appositional bone from undue stress
      c. Disturbance of local organizer or variation in vascular supply

D. Contour
  1. Formation and remodeling of bone
  2. Abnormalities
      a. Excess tubulation: thin shaft
          (1) Poor muscular development
          (2) Systemic mesenchymal disease
      b. Excess cortical bone: flaring of shaft
          (1) Excess focal response to injury
          (2) Acromegaly
          (3) Degenerative change
          (4) Tumor
          (5) Subperiosteal new bone from periosteal elevation
      c. Bowing in bone softening process
      d. Internal expansion
          (1) Focal widening: expanding intramedullary lesion
          (2) Generalized widening: general effect on forming bone

E. Configuration (combined abnormalities)
  1. Aseptic necrosis—density, size, contour, focus
  2. Tumor—density, size, contour, number involved bones
  3. Infection—density, contour, number involved bones

F. Location
  1. Significant in fractures and dislocations (right-angle and special oblique views may be necessary)
  2. Dislocations difficult to detect roentgenographically if portions of bone still cartilaginous

G. Number
  1. Increased: polydactylism
  2. Decreased: phocomelia, posttraumatic amputation, destructive disease

H. Margination
  1. Normal: distinctness of trabecular pattern, cortical margins
  2. Reduced (resorption of calcium in subperiosteal area)
      a. Inflammatory disease of soft tissues or bone
      b. Metabolic disturbance: calcium mobilized from bone (e.g., hyperparathyroidism)
      c. Elevation of periosteum by hemorrhage or tumor
      d. Resorption of bony fragment edges at fracture margins as part of healing process

The principles outlined in the preceding chapters are valid in examining the appendicular areas. Roentgenographically these areas contain three components: soft, articular, and skeletal (osseous) tissues.

SOFT TISSUE COMPONENT

The soft tissue components (skin, fat, muscles, fascia, ligaments, lymphatics, and blood vessels) vary in amount and density. The normality or abnormality of these components is detected by using these parameters.

The primary naturally occurring contrast used to delineate the soft tissue structures is the radiolucency of the fat. Fat is found in the subcutaneous tissues, between the muscle bundles, and around joints. Good quality radiographs of the arms and legs demonstrate the soft tissue components with the fat appearing ra-

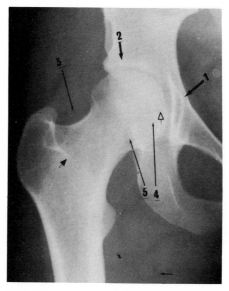

Fig. 3-1. Roentgenographic examination of the osseous structures, joints, and soft tissues requires recognition of all these structures. In this A-P view of a normal hip the floor of the acetabulum is identified (*1*). This is the depression in the floor of the acetabulum which lies between the horseshoe shaped, densely corticated, articulating surfaces. Within the depth of this recess is the fat pad called the pulvinar. The weight bearing surface of the acetabulum (*2*) lies superiorly and is routinely denser. The insertion of the ligamentum teres into the femoral head occurs at the fovea capitalis (open arrow). The margin of the capsule of the hip joint is set off by a radiolucent line of fat (*3*). At the point of the solid arrow (*3*) there is thickening of the capsule to produce the zona orbicularis. This is the lateral neck of the capsule, although some prolongation extends more laterally. This also marks the area of approximate penetration of the retinacular vessels. The anterior (*4*) and posterior (*5*) margins of the acetabulum are identified as white lines crossing the femoral head. A rather faint white line crosses the base of the femoral neck representing the intertrochanteric crest (short tailed arrow) which lies on the posterior surface of the femur and represents the most lateral extent of the capsule posteriorly. The small lower arrow indicates the fat line between the muscles of the thigh. The articular cartilage of the hip occupies the distance between the weight bearing surface (*2*) and the appositional surface of the femoral head.

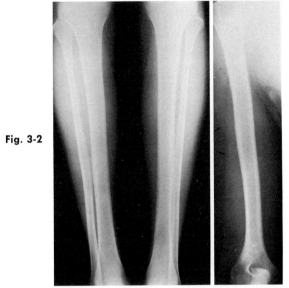

Fig. 3-2   Fig. 3-3

Fig. 3-2. This view of the calves of the legs shows the normal muscle masses with the skin edge defined against the air. The shape, density, and cortical thickness of the tibias and fibulas are normal.

Fig. 3-3. The muscle masses of the arm are well set off (solid arrows) against the subcutaneous fat. The structure of the humerus is normal.

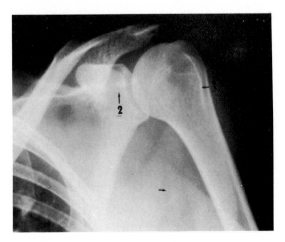

Fig. 3-4. The film of the shoulder shows the relationship of the humeral head to the glenoid fossa of the scapula. The superior margin is represented by the acromion of the scapula with the anterior margin shown by the coracoid process (2) overlying the glenoid fossa. Along the anterolateral aspect of the humerus is the bicipital groove (1), bounded by the greater and lesser tuberosities. The soft tissue fat lines (solid arrow) are set off between the skin folds and the muscle masses about the shoulder.

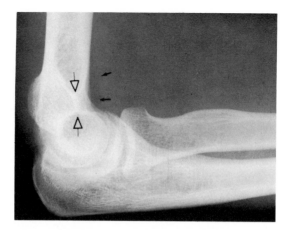

Fig. 3-5. The lateral view of the elbow joint shows the anterior and posterior humeral fossae of the distal humerus identified as a solid white cortical line (apposing open arrows). Lying in these fossae are fat pads. The anterior fat pad is normally seen (solid arrows). The fossae allow the olecranon process and conoid process to ride further inward into the humerus during extension and flexion. Displacement of the fat pad occurs with joint effusion.

Fig. 3-6

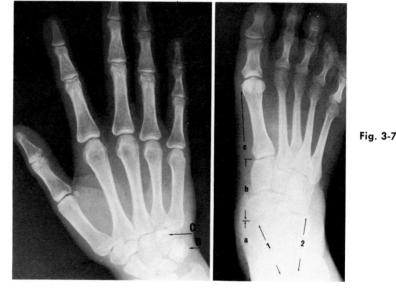

Fig. 3-7

Fig. 3-6. This view of a normal adult hand shows fat lines paralleling the proximal phalanges (*B*) in contrast to the soft tissue irregularities representing knuckle folds (*A*). The osseous structures in the wrist show a normal appearance. The hook of the hamate (*C*) projects through the body of the hamate. The pisiform is somewhat hidden by the triquetrum, but its margins are identified (*D*).

Fig. 3-7. Normal adult foot. Bony density and the alignment of the components of the foot are normal. The forefoot (*c*) is composed of the metatarsals and phalanges. There is normally some tendency to varus alignment of the first metatarsal. The midfoot (*b*) is composed of five of the tarsals. The hindfoot (*a*) articulates with the midfoot at the junction of the talus (*1*), the navicular, the calcaneus (*2*), and the cuboid. The angle formed between the calcaneus and the talus is normal. Specific types of abnormality produce changes in this angle.

diolucent or darker grey than the muscles or adjoining ligaments. Changes may occur in the fat deposit—an obese individual may show extensive fatty deposits in the subcutaneous areas and between the muscle bundles while a thin individual may have small fatty deposits (Figs. 3-1 to 3-7).

Abnormal naturally occurring radiopacities usually represent excess calcium deposits. The most frequent site of such deposits is in the blood vessels. For example, it is common to find calcific deposits along the course of the arteries of the thighs. Calcium deposit in the arterial wall, disproportionate to the patient's age, occurs in some systemic diseases such as hyperparathyroidism and diabetes mellitus (Fig. 3-8). The veins or lymphatics may contain calcium deposits (phleboliths), particularly if the channels are broad. Sometimes, the calcific deposits represent ectopic bone formation, as in patients with varicose veins, hematoma from repeated trauma, or burns. Venous and lymphatic tumors (angioma and lymphangiomas) are predisposed to phlebolith deposits (Fig. 3-9). Subcutaneous calcification can occur with certain systemic diseases such as scleroderma and dermatomyositis (Fig. 3-10).

Better definition of the soft tissue structures is obtained by changing the roentgenographic contrast between adjoining structures (Fig. 3-11). Opacification of arteries, veins, and lymphatics of the extremities (arteriography, venography, lymphangiography) permits the detection of intrinsic disease (aneurysm, tumor,

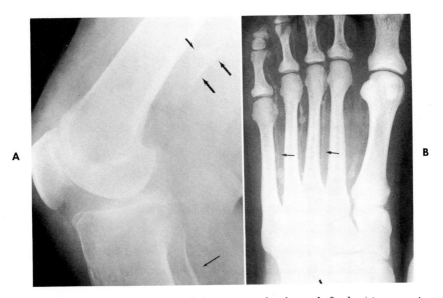

Fig. 3-8. A, Naturally occurring increased densities result when calcific deposits occur in arterial walls as the result of atheromatous change. The broad arrows indicate femoral artery calcification; the artery is somewhat dilated. The lower arrow shows similar calcifications in the arteries of the calf. At the margins of the articulating surfaces of the knee bony overgrowth indicates senescent joint change. **B,** Marked deposit of calcium along the course of the arteries is shown. The interdigital arteries (small arrow) are extensively calcified. This occurs in individuals with diabetes or with disturbance of calcium metabolism, as in this patient with hyperparathyroidism.

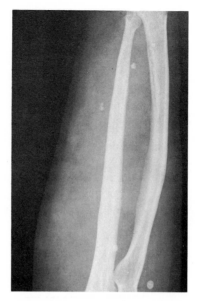

Fig. 3-9. Irregular distortion of soft tissues, irregular bony overgrowth of the radius, and multiple calcific densities within the soft tissues all demonstrate the presence of a vascular tumor. Abnormalities are reflected by change in size, density, and configuration.

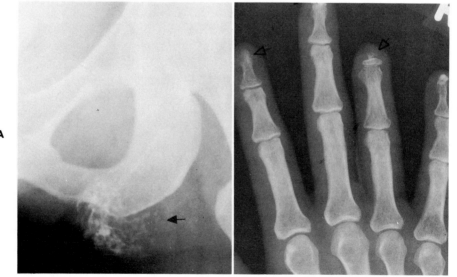

Fig. 3-10. A, Irregular calcifications have occurred in the soft tissues in the region of the bursa (arrow). This irregularly linear calcific deposit occurs in collagen disease, in this case, scleroderma. B, Irregular soft tissue calcifications in the tip of the phalanges (solid arrow) also results from scleroderma. There is also deformity and loss of density of the terminal tufts of the fingers (left open arrow) involving the second digit. In contrast, the distal phalanx of the fourth digit (right open arrow) is almost completely absent as the result of early traumatic amputation.

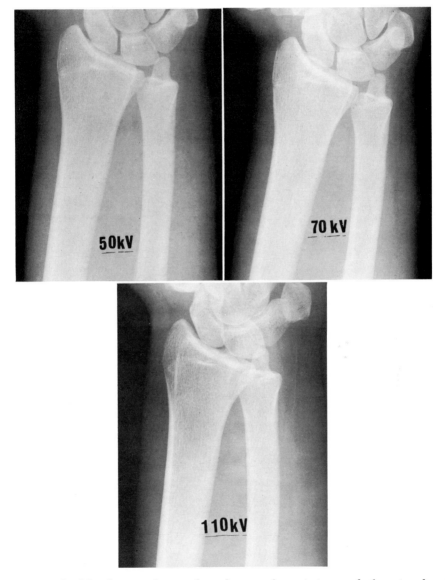

Fig. 3-11. As the kilovoltage used to produce the x-ray beam is increased, there is a loss in definition of the small bony trabeculae and of the soft tissue planes. This results from the production of a more penetrating beam, less of which is absorbed by the small osseous and soft tissue structures.

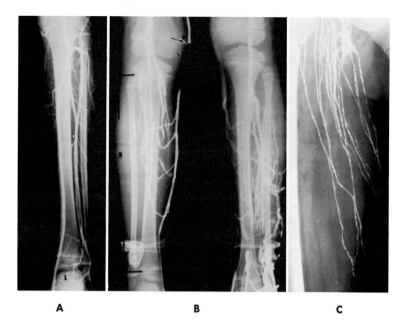

A   **B**   **C**

Fig. 3-12. **A,** Injection of an iodinated compound into the femoral artery produces opacification of the arteries of this normal lower leg. **B,** Injection of contrast medium into the veins when the veins are compressed by a tourniquet shows filling of the venous system. The valves of the vein (*v*), which prevent reflux, are seen. The right tibia (*R*) is shorter than the left as the result of overgrowth from excess vascularity on the left. **C,** The normal lymphatic channels in the thigh are filled with contrast material. The filling is rather irregular since the medium is oily and forms droplets.

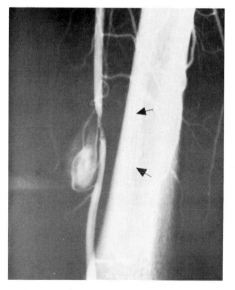

Fig. 3-13. Injection of an iodinated compound into a brachial artery shows opacification of the more distal portions of the artery. There is escape of the contrast medium into a small sac, a traumatic aneurysm. Collateral circulation is observed (solid arrows). Change of contrast permits definitive diagnosis.

rupture, etc.) or obstruction or distortion by extrinsic disease (Figs. 3-12 and 3-13).

Abnormal spaces may be present in the soft tissue. Such spaces are usually sinus tracts or communications from a pocket of infection or along the course of a penetrating object such as a bullet. If the sinuses reach the skin, iodinated compounds injected through the openings can define their extent and the location. This is helpful in the treatment of chronic infection.

The size of the individual structures or the amount of individual tissue is indicative of normality. Dilatation of the blood vessels as in aneurysm or tumor is an example of a variation in size. Excess fat deposit can occur with muscular atrophy or fatty tumors (Fig. 3-14). Reduction of fat may be seen in individuals suffering from malnutrition. Certain systemic diseases produce an abnormality by edema that causes the fat to appear decreased since there is less radiolucency. Excess soft tissue in the subcutaneous areas may be noted in some metabolic disorders such as myxedema (hypothyroidism) or acromegaly, which produces a thickening of the tissues of the heel pad (Figs. 3-15 and 3-16).

Collections of abnormal tissue such as tumors or hematomas may cause apparent increase in size of muscle masses (Figs. 3-17 and 3-18). Comparison with films of the opposite extremity makes it easier to detect these individual variations.

Decreased amount or size of soft tissues in focal views is found with surgical removal, fat necrosis, congenital absence of muscular development, or disuse.

The known aids in determining the causes behind alteration in size of soft tissues are as follows: Increased size of muscles as the result of tumor is usually

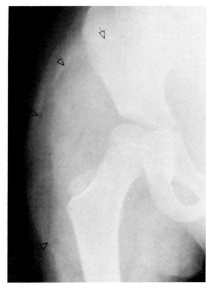

Fig. 3-14. Reduced radiodensity may occur naturally. A large radiolucent mass overlies. the right hip (arrows). This represents a fatty tumor (liposarcoma) of the buttocks.

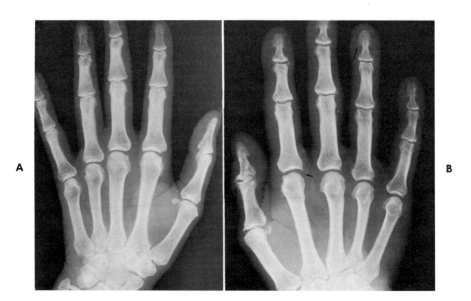

Fig. 3-15. **A,** A normal adult female hand. **B,** The hand of a woman with acromegaly (hyper-activity of the anterior lobe of the pituitary). Bony overgrowth occurs about the terminal tuft (small arrow). Accentuated degenerative change is noted around the interphalangeal and metacarpal phalangeal joints of the thumb. The articular cartilage is thickened (small arrow) as seen in the metacarpal phalangeal joint of the second digit.

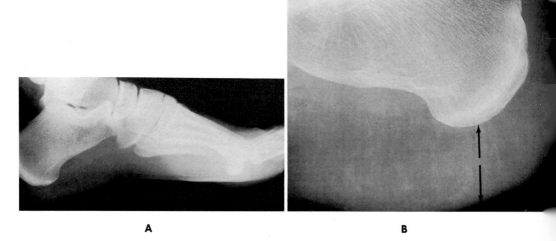

Fig. 3-16. **A,** A normal lateral view of the foot. Notice the distance between the base of the os calcis and the heel pad in the normal foot. **B,** The relative thickness of the heel pad is increased (arrows); such increase is the result of acromegaly if it exceeds 25 mm.

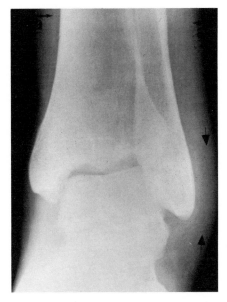

Fig. 3-17. Definition of the soft tissues may be lost as the result of edema. Following a twisting injury to the ankle the soft tissues overlying the lateral malleolus (apposing solid arrows) are exceptionally prominent; there is loss of definition of the fat lines. The medial subcutaneous fat (*a*, double-ended arrow) is undisturbed, whereas the lateral fat line (*a*, single pointed arrow) shows loss of definition and distortion as the result of the edema.

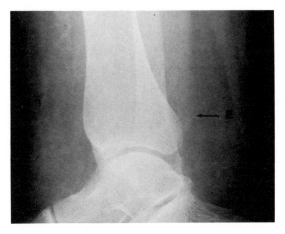

Fig. 3-18. Obstruction of lymphatics produces lymphedema. The distance from the muscle mass to the skin (*a*) is markedly increased, and dilated lymyphatic channels (small solid arrows) extend throughout the subcutaneous fat and blur the margin of the muscle masses.

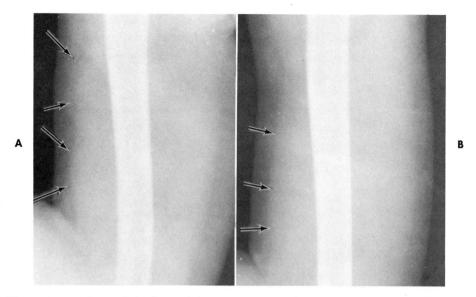

Fig. 3-19. Irregularity of the form of the muscle may result from intrinsic disease. **A,** At the time of birth the long head of the biceps muscle was ruptured (arrows). The biceps muscle is bunched in the midportion of the arm as a result of the rupture. **B,** The normal side shows a smooth margin of the muscle mass.

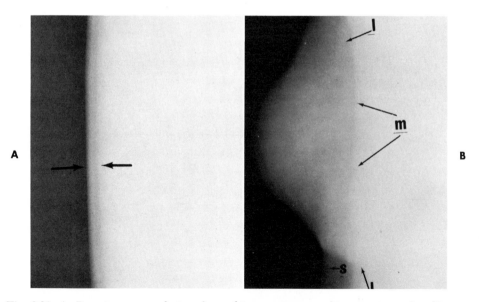

Fig. 3-20. A, By using proper factors for making roentgenographic exposures, the skin can be easily seen. The outer arrow points to the surface of the skin; the inner arrow points to the subcutaneous fat. The soft tissue density lying between the outer arrow and the fat represents the thickness of the skin. This is normal. **B,** In contrast, a soft tissue mass (lipoma) projects posteriorly from the thigh, with the edges of the muscle mass (*m*) in apposition to the margins of the lipoma (upper and lower *l*). The skin (*s*) can be identified; its margination is poorly defined at the edge of the mass.

accompanied by distortion of the normal configuration; sharp margination may be lost. Rupture of the tendinous insertion of a muscle causes contraction to an abnormal degree, producing a "bunching" of a muscle mass (Fig. 3-19). The muscle will appear to have increased in size, but in actuality the thickness has increased while the length has decreased. Blood vessels undergoing degeneration as a result of age provide the most frequent distortion of normal contour of the soft tissues; there is both dilatation and tortuosity. Full appreciation of this configuration requires contrast injection into the vessel.

Alteration of the definition and thickness of the skin from pressure, overgrowth, small tumors, or edema can be identified roentgenographically. The extremities are in essence cylinders; therefore, in order to detect an abnormality of the skin it is necessary to view it tangentially (Fig. 3-20). Films of the extremity taken at various angles may be needed in order to adequately localize a roentgenographic finding.

The ability to predict the normal location of blood vessels and lymphatics of the extremities makes possible the use of these structures as a guide for normality. Ligaments, tendons, and muscle masses, however, may also be displaced by tumor or other excess soft tissue. More careful viewing of the films is needed to detect this abnormality. If there is dislocation of a joint, the soft tissues appear malaligned when compared to the opposite side.

Increase in the number of blood vessels occurs with tumors, particularly malignant tumors (Fig. 3-21). The blood vessels in tumors are abnormal both in

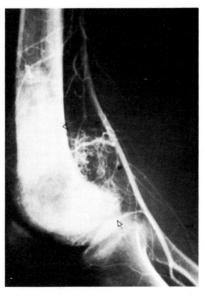

Fig. 3-21. Naturally occurring increased density of the bone coupled with expansion and irregularity of contour of the bone occurs with tumors such as osteogenic sarcoma. This tumor, in addition, shows excess blood vessels, opacified by arterial injection (open arrows). The mass has displaced the popliteal artery (solid arrows) posteriorly.

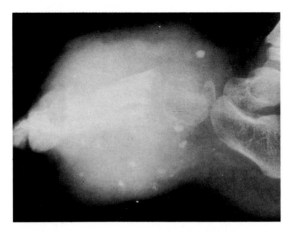

Fig. 3-22. A massive hemangioma of the foot has caused distortion of bone as well as extensive calcification.

configuration and location. Vascular malformation, such as angiomas, or collateral circulation from obstruction of a major artery may be demonstrated (Fig. 3-22). A decreased number of blood vessels may also be observed with obstruction, since many of the small vessels may not fill.

Since definition of the margins of the muscles and the soft tissues is dependent upon fat, anything that will either reduce the fat or distort it, such as edema, inflammation, or tumor, will decrease the sharpness of the margins of the soft tissue structures.

ARTICULAR COMPONENT

The joints of the extremities allow mobility of the osseous components and in part are a portion of the osseous structures. The soft tissue components of the articulations must also be considered when the roentgenograms are viewed. The margins of the joint capsule, synovial lining, articular cartilage, and adjoining ligaments and tendons are partly identifiable when contrasted to adjacent structures (Fig. 3-23). The distance between the articulating margins of adjoining bones indicates the thickness of the articular cartilage. The subcutaneous and periarticular fat permits the edges of other soft tissue structures of the joints to be identified. The positive contrast of the calcium in the bone and the negative contrast of the radiolucency of the fat allow direct or indirect roentgenographic demonstration of the various structures.

Variations of density may occur normally; the most frequent is soft tissue calcification. This is usually deposited on the margins of the tendons (peritendonitis calcarea) and may later rupture into an adjoining bursa (Fig. 3-24). Degenerative change of the capsules also produces minor excess calcific deposits or excess bone formation at the capsular insertion (Fig. 3-25). Calcification or degeneration occurs as well in articular cartilages or menisci such as the knee joint (Fig. 3-26). Hemorrhage, tumor, or metabolic disturbance (gout) may

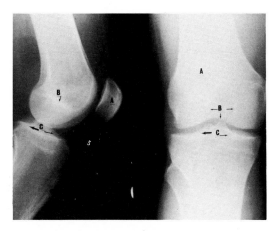

Fig. 3-23. The lateral and A-P roentgenograms of the knee utilize the contrast of bone, soft tissue, and fat to show anatomic structures. The patella (*A*) lies between the patellar grooves of the anterior aspect of the femur. The intercondylar notch (*B*) is well visualized in the A-P projection. On the lateral projection it can be seen as a dense white line (*B*). The intercondylar eminence provides the origin for the base of the cruciate ligaments (*C*). The small arrow pointing anteriorly and medially represents the site of insertion of the anterior cruciate whereas the broader arrow represents the site of origin of the posterior cruciate ligament. Overlying the anterior aspect of the tibia on the lateral projection is the tibial tubercle (*4*) into which the patellar ligament (*3*) inserts. The suprapatellar fat pad (*2*) lies above the patella and deep to the gastrocnemius tendon (*1*).

appear as periarticular soft tissue calcification. On occasion, the joint space itself becomes radiolucent from spontaneous formation of intra-articular gas (Fig. 3-27). A sharp decrease in the pressure within the joint permits the fluid in the joint to vaporize, causing the radiolucency (vacuum phenomenon). When such an event occurs, it is possible to identify definitively the thickness of portions of the articular cartilages and study the joint space itself. Arthrography is the injection of a contrast medium, either positive contrast (iodinated compounds) or negative contrast (air), and the recording of the appearance of the joint on roentgenograms (Fig. 3-28). When air is injected the appearance is similar to that seen as a result of a vacuum phenomenon. The smallness of the joint space is somewhat surprising, since frequently one forgets the thickness of the articular cartilages when viewing plain films. The various outpocketings (bursae) that communicate with the joint space of the various articulations also fill with the medium and can be shown on roentgenograms. Excess filling or failure of a bursa to fill may indicate abnormality (Fig. 3-29). Comparison of the opposite extremity will help in determining thickness of articular cartilage of a joint. This distance may appear to be increased with dislocation, by effusion, or with thickening of the cartilage in acromegaly (Fig. 3-30). The most frequent abnormality is a decreased distance between the articulating margins of the osseous structures. The cartilaginous thickness is reduced, usually by degeneration but occasionally as a result of postinflammatory or posttraumatic destruction. After surgical removal of portions of the articular cartilage or of the meniscus

Text continued on p. 164.

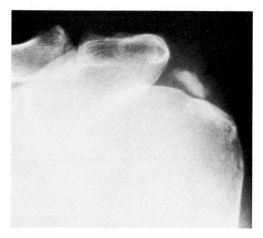

Fig. 3-24. Abnormal density may result from excess calcium deposit in the soft tissues, such as the subdeltoid bursa above the greater tuberosity of the humerus (solid arrow). This is a common abnormality around joints and may result from trauma, infection, or unknown causes.

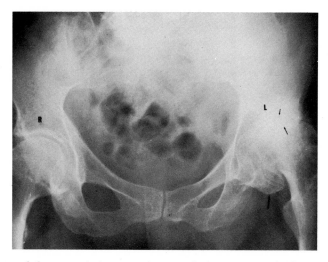

Fig. 3-25. Increased density and change in form result from attritional (degenerative) change. The left hip shows severe loss of cartilage, with increased density at the weight bearing surface between the femur and the acetabulum. There is bony overgrowth below the acetabulum (broad arrow) and superior and lateral to the acetabulum (small arrows). This represents advanced degenerative change.

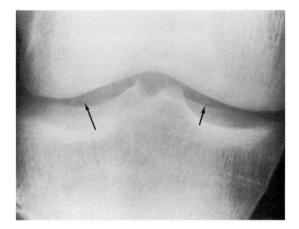

Fig. 3-26. Minute calcifications (arrows) are present in the menisci as the result of degenerative change in the cartilaginous structure. This is a less common finding than calcific bursitis.

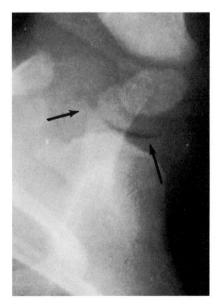

Fig. 3-27. Reduction in density may occur spontaneously in a normal joint. The crescentic radiolucency between the solid arrows represents gas formed under the influence of negative pressure in the shoulder of an 18-month-old child. The distance between the margins of the crescent indicate the width of the joint space—the distance between the articular cartilage of the humeral head and the articular cartilage of the glenoid fossa of the scapula.

A   **B**

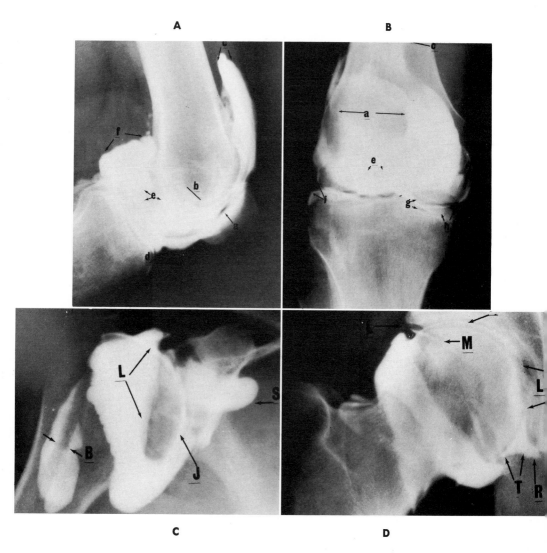

C   **D**

Fig. 3-28. For legend see opposite page.

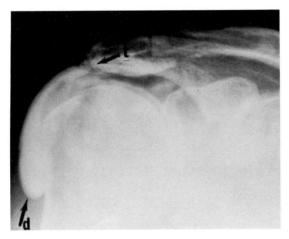

Fig. 3-29. Disruption of continuity of the rotator cuff (*t*) allows excess extension of the contrast medium along the course of the bicipital groove (*d*) with excess filling of the subdeltoid bursa. The joint space, however, is still opacified.

Fig. 3-28. Injection of an iodinated compound into the joint spaces demonstrates the internal structures. **A,** Lateral view of the knee. The upper margin of the suprapatellar bursa (*c*) is the site of its muscle attachment. The retropatellar area (*a*) shows the thickness of the articular cartilage. The intercondylar notch (*b*) defines the superior margin of the joint space. The cruciate ligaments cross in the central portion of the joint (*e*). The anterior ligament (small arrow) is relaxed; the posterior ligament (double arrow) is under stretch. The intercondylar eminence lies below (*e*), and is obscured by the contrast medium. The posterior portion of the joint space (*f*) distends with the knee flexed. Anteriorly the transverse ligament between the menisci (*d*) encroaches on the contrast medium. **B,** A-P projection. The patella (*a*) is surrounded by contrast medium. The cruciate ligaments (*e*) are obscured by contrast medium. The suprapatellar bursa (*c*) is seen as a thin tongue of contrast medium. The articular cartilages (*g*) are defined against thin layers of contrast medium. The medial meniscus (*h*) is a triangular radiolucency, broad medially and tapering toward the central portion of the joint. The lateral meniscus (*i*) is more irregular since it is not attached to the femoral fibular ligament; the contrast medium, therefore, collects between the lateral margin of the meniscus and the ligament. This is in contrast to the femoral tibial ligament which closely invests the medial aspect of the medial meniscus. **C,** The internal structure of the shoulder. The joint space (*J*) lies between the articular cartilage of the humerus and the scapula. The labrum of the glenoid fossa (*L*) is cartilaginous and not seen on the routine film; it is shown when contrast medium is injected. The subacromial bursa (*S*) is somewhat small. The tendon of the long head of the biceps (*B*) is outlined by contrast medium extending along the course of the bicipital groove. **D,** Arthrography of the hip joint. The joint space (upper arrow) is thin. The ligamentum teres (*LT*) is set off by contrast medium as it reaches the fovea capitalis. The transverse ligament (*T*) elevates the joint capsule, setting off the acetabular recesses (*R*) which lie on either side of the ligamentum teres and above the transverse ligament. The anterior margin of the acetabulum (*M*) shows a fine radiolucent line next to a thin layer of contrast medium anterior to the femoral head and neck. The labrum of the articular cartilage (*L*) extends beyond the margin of the bony acetabulum. Laterally the zona orbicularis (*O*) is seen as a broad band of radiolucency that interrupts the opacification of the capsule laterally.

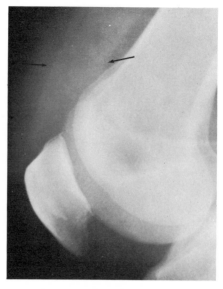

Fig. 3-30. Joint effusion is manifested by distention of bursae. One of the classic areas for this is in the knee. The suprapatellar bursa (apposing solid arrows) demonstrates the dilatation of this bursa in contrast to the normal knee.

Fig. 3-31

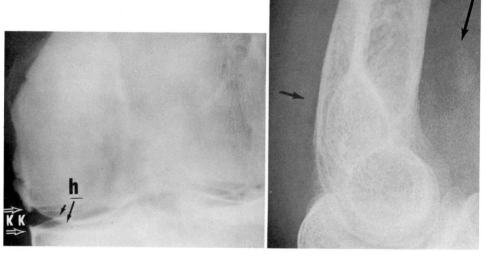

Fig. 3-31. Arthrography may also show derangement of internal anatomy not detactable on routine films. The medial meniscus (*h*) shows extension of the contrast medium into the body of the meniscus (*k*-arrows) as the result of a tear from trauma.

Fig. 3-32. Effusion in the elbow joint may cause displacement of the fat pad in the humeral fossae. The anterior fat pad (long arrow) is extruded completely from the shallow fossa. This fat pad is normally partially visible. The posterior fat pad (short arrow) is not seen unless joint effusion has intervened. A fracture of the head of the radius caused the effusion.

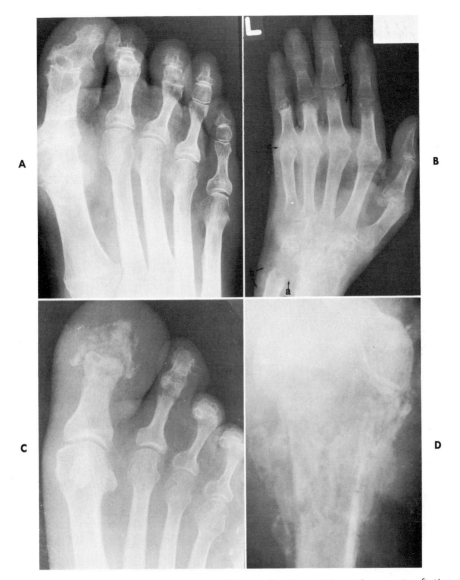

Fig. 3-33. Bony and periarticular destruction changes density and form. Increased soft tissues result from a variety of disease processes. **A,** Gout produces periarticular punched out lesions with extensive adjoining soft tissue masses that may calcify. The bony density of the osseous structures generally is not appreciably reduced. **B,** In contrast, rheumatoid arthritis causes diffuse demineralization of the osseous structures. Erosions, rather than punched out lesions, involve the ulnar-radial (*a*) articulation of the wrist; soft tissue swelling (representing rheumatoid nodule) overlying the ulnar styloid (*b*); loss of cartilage and joint effusion at the metacarpal phalangeal articulation (*c*); and most characteristic loss of the proximal interphalangeal articulations (*d*). The severe loss of cartilage is also characteristic of advanced rheumatoid arthritis, with subluxations occurring at the metacarpal phalangeal articulations. **C,** Focal inflammatory disease (osteomyelitis) may destroy bone, causing expansion and soft tissue swelling. Staphylococcus osteomyelitis produces these changes. The other osseous structures are not severely affected. **D,** Prolonged inflammatory disease (*d*) produces irregular soft tissue calcifications and new bone formation (involucrum) surrounding the shaft of the proximal humerus. The remaining undestroyed cortex (sequestra) lie within the involucrum. Openings passing from the medullary cavity to the outer portion of the involucrum (cloaca) are identifiable.

of the knee, closer apposition of the articulating margins of the bones can be seen.

The irregularity found in degeneration or in posttraumatic state is usually insufficient to detect even with arthrography. One exception is the meniscus of the knee, where tears of the cartilage can be demonstrated by arthrography (Fig. 3-31). Severe loss of cartilage, causing irregular surfaces, can occasionally be demonstrated. Excess fluid within the joint produces distention of the joint capsule and bursae. The finding of a distorted bursa can be identified on routine roentgenograms if one knows the appearance of the normal joint. Two useful examples are the knee and the elbow. When there is joint effusion in the knee, the suprapatellar bursa distends, occluding the retropatellar fat pad. When there is excess fluid in the elbow, displacement of the anterior and posterior fat pads of the humerus occurs (Fig. 3-32). Distinctness of margination is dependent upon outlining of the soft tissues by fat. The causes for loss of radiolucency of fat, edema, fluid, and inflammatory infiltrate all pertain to the joints as well. Loss of definition of the bony margin of the joint may result from infection, inflammation, disuse, or hyperemia (Fig. 3-33).

SKELETAL COMPONENTS

The most frequent reason for roentgenographic examination of the extremities is to detect abnormality from trauma. Identification of a fracture line may be very difficult, depending upon the degree of mineralization of the bone, the severity of the fracture, and the bone which is involved (Figs. 3-34 to 3-36). Finding a fracture may be easier than assessing the status of bone. The long bone should be considered as composed of several components. The epiphyseal cartilage in youth is seen as a radiolucent stripe crossing the ends of the bone. Epiphyseal ossification centers develop beyond the epiphyseal cartilage within the ends of the bone. These appear at a predictable age and allow determination of the skeletal age (Fig. 3-37). The rate and degree of bodily maturation can be judged when compared to predicted standards for the number of epiphyseal centers that should be present at a given age. The metaphysis represents the most rapidly growing portion of the bone. The diaphysis comprises the major portion of the body of the bone. The bone, on cross section, shows an outer cortex covered on its outer surface with periosteum and an inner layer of endosteum. The central cavity of the bone contains the medullary tissue and the spongiosa. Certain diseases selectively affect any of these individual areas. Identification of the appearance of the various components is needed to understand and interpret roentgenograms of the appendicular skeleton. The structure of the bone reveals systemic status and metabolic status, and therefore, provides an excellent indicator of calcium and phosphorus metabolism and reflects many of the hormonal states. Prolonged stress produces variation in form or density of bone, indicating how the body has functioned mechanically in the past (Fig. 3-38). If the various parameters outlined in the preceding sections are followed in viewing roentgenograms of the osseous structures, accurate categorization of diseases and diagnoses can be made (Fig. 3-39).

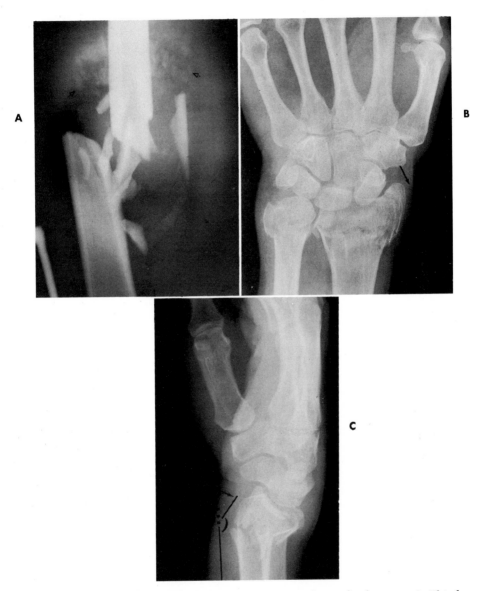

Fig. 3-34. Fractures represent discontinuity of the cortex as the result of trauma. **A,** This fracture of the femur produces gross fragmentation of the shaft. Callus deposit (open arrows) is occurring about the fracture. Markedly abnormal alignment of the femoral shaft and the fracture fragments is present. **B,** In the A-P projection of the wrist, the comminution of the distal shaft of the radius and ulna is observed; the fracture fragments are impacted; that is, one fragment is compressed into the other. The radial styloid (solid arrow) has been displaced toward the thumb and toward the elbow. On the lateral projection (**C**) it can be seen that the articulating surface of the radius has been angled dorsally. The degree of angulation (arrow, solid lines) is apparent with the dotted line demonstrating the usual alignment of the radius. This is called the silver fork deformity of the wrist, and the angulation produces severe dysfunction.

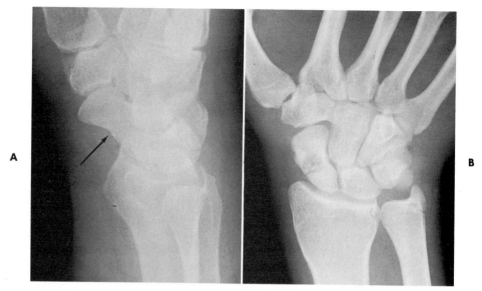

A

B

Fig. 3-35. A, A small linear fracture of the carpal navicular (solid arrow) is difficult to demonstrate unless the proper films are taken. This fracture may fail to heal. **B,** Bony resorption may occur about the fracture site, producing the rounded radiolucency. The body of the navicular bone is increased in density as the result of interruption of the blood supply (ischemic necrosis). A similar finding may occur in the femoral head with fracture of the femoral neck.

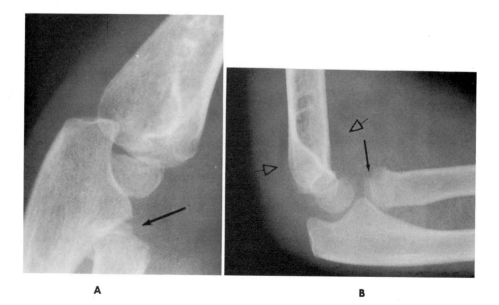

A

B

Fig. 3-36. Epiphyseal fractures occur in children. The secondary epiphyseal center for the proximal end of the radius (solid arrow) is seen in the oblique projection (**A**) and in the lateral projection (**B**). The epiphyseal plate has been disrupted. The fracture involves the elbow joint; the anterior and posterior fat pads (open arrows) have been displaced out of their usual fossae in the distal humerus.

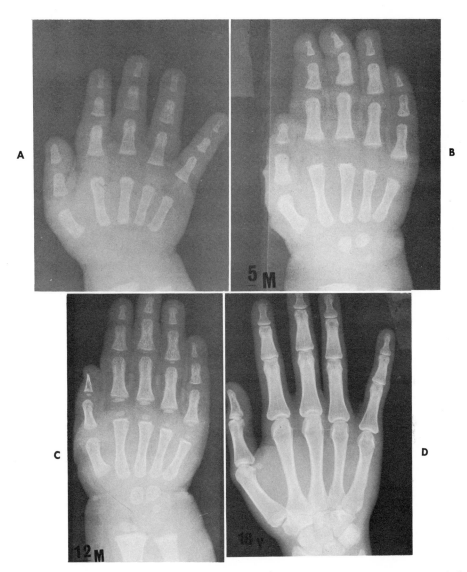

Fig. 3-37. There is a predictable pattern in the development of the bony structures of the hand and wrist. The number and configuration of the bony structures provide a guide for normal bony development. **A,** The newborn's hand shows none of the secondary centers for the wrist. **B,** By the end of 5 months centers are developing in the wrist and beginning to appear at the distal ends of the metacarpals. **C,** By the end of 12 months there is development of the epiphysis of the distal end of the radius; the centers for the phalanges are also noted. The maturation of the wrist, in this instance, approximates two years and the phalanges 15 months. Such discrepancies are fairly common. **D,** In adulthood the secondary centers have developed and fused to the adjoining primary centers, and the form of the centers is now that of an adult. Detailed atlases are available demonstrating centers of development for all of the childhood and adolescent periods.

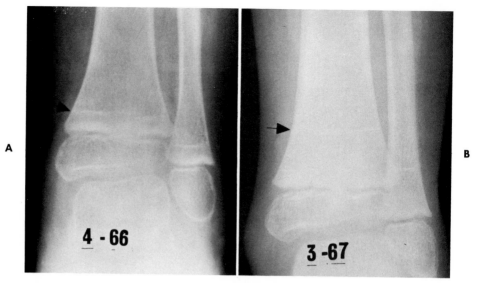

Fig. 3-38. Linear increased densities are commonly seen in the shafts of long bones (growth lines). These usually reflect either systemic disease or injury. **A,** The growth line in April of 1966 (solid arrow) lies fairly close to the epiphyseal cartilage of the distal tibia. **B,** Approximately a year later the growth line lies further from the end of the shaft of the tibia, indicating growth of the length of the bone at the epiphyseal cartilage. The growth rate of the tibia in this case may have been accentuated somewhat by the injury to the leg.

Density. While the trabeculae of the medullary cavity can be seen, the cortex of the bone contains more calcium, making it the denser of the two. Because bones are tubular, two layers of cortex are usually superimposed upon the medullary cavity. When the beam is projected tangentially to the bone, as on the edge of a bone, it becomes very dense. Increase in thickness of the cortex, as in response to unusual stress, may cause even greater radiodensity. Excess deposits of calcium in an abnormal pattern occur in certain diseases (osteosclerosis). No attempt will be made in this text to list the multiple causes for this condition. Metastatic disease, bone islands, Paget's disease, residual excess cortical bone from healed fractures or infection, and abnormal stress are the most common causes for an increased density. Identification of the part of the bone which has increased density (periosteal bone deposit, endosteal bone deposit, trabeculae) aids in differentiating diseases or stress. Comparison of the opposite limbs is necessary for the next step in evaluation of increased density—determining if the density is a focal hyperdensity, a local hyperdensity—confined to one bone— a total unilateral hyperdensity, or a total systemic hyperdensity (Fig. 3-40).

Decreased density, a much more frequent abnormality, indicates reduced calcium deposits and may result from bone resorption, failure of new bone formation, or replacement of bone by other tissues. Failure of matrix formation prevents calcium deposit in the bone (osteoporosis) and frequently occurs in postmenopausal women. Next to degenerative changes, osteoporosis is the most

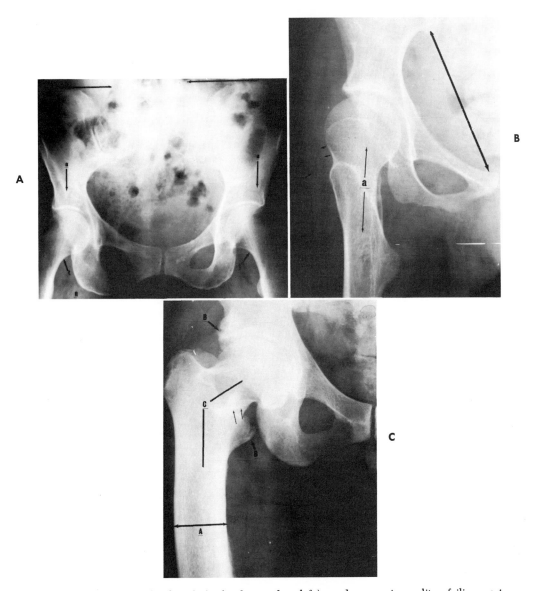

Fig. 3-39. A, Unequal leg length (right shorter than left) produces an inequality of iliac crest height (broad lines, right being lower than left). The supporting trabeculae above the right hip (a) are increased in number, compared to the left, and are indicative of the unusual stress. The lateral margin of the right acetabulum has also increased somewhat to give added lateral support. The trabecula of the femoral neck (t) also shows the stress response, with the right being greater than the left. B, Lack of muscle power from neurologic deficit produces bony deformity. The femoral neck is very straight (a), representing a valgus alignment. The shaft of the femur is thinned (apposing solid arrows). The muscle masses are poorly developed and there is excess fat in the soft tissues (small arrows). The pelvis is small and somewhat deformed (broad, double-ended arrow). C, Abnormal consistency of the bone at an early age may change size and form of the adult bone. The femoral neck shows varus alignment (C). There is bony overgrowth about the lesser trochanter (B) and about the superior aspect of the acetabulum (B). These represent bony overgrowth as the result of abnormal stress. A healed incomplete fracture through the femoral neck (small arrows) is identified as a linear increased density. The width of the femoral shaft is increased (A) indicated by the double-ended arrow. This individual suffered from renal rickets with bone softening at an early age, and the changes result from abnormal alignment of the osseous structures.

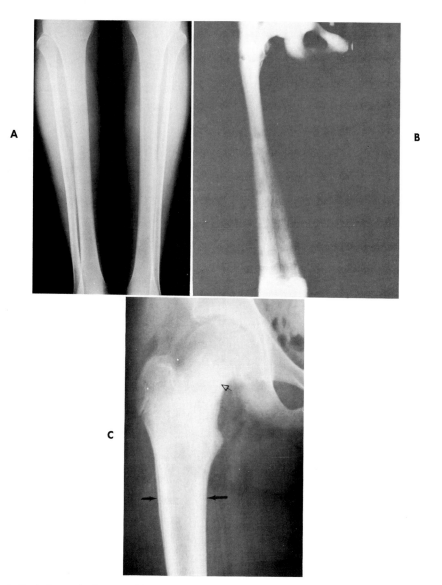

Fig. 3-40. A, Normal tibia and fibula. Note definition of the medullary cavity and relative cortical thickness. **B,** Osteopetrosis; the femur is club-shaped, the medullary cavity obliterated, and the density diffusely increased with incomplete fracture. **C,** Ewing's sarcoma; periosteal new bone (apposing solid arrows), increased density of the medullary cavity (open arrow), and loss of cortex (open arrow). **D,** Paget's disease; irregular accentuated trabeculae are in the medullary cavity with bowing, and thick cortex. **E,** Pulmonary hypertrophic osteoarthropathy; cortical thickening of the fibula and tibia (lower arrows) with increased diameter of the fibular shaft (double-ended arrows); the medullary cavity is unaffected. **F,** Healed osteomyelitis with sequestrum formation (small arrow); loss of normal cortical contour, irregular density in the medullary cavity, with thickened shaft.

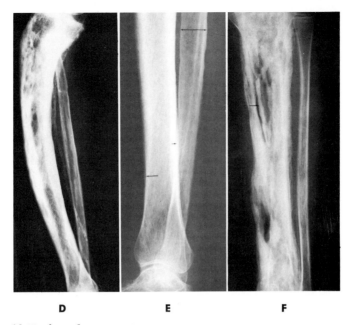

D   E   F

Fig. 3-40, cont'd. For legend see opposite page.

common systemic abnormality detected. Lack of sufficient calcium to ossify formed matrix (osteomalacia) may reflect disturbance of calcium absorption from the intestinal tract or excessive bodily demand for calcium, as in hyperparathyroidism, primary or secondary. Acute systemic processes which affect bone are reflected in the most metabolically active portion of the bone, which, in the growing bone, is the metaphysis. Thus, rickets (osteomalacia) is noted at the metaphyses (Fig. 3-41). Changes in density are most frequently seen in the region of the knee, the wrist, and the ankle. Transverse lines of increased density across the shaft of the bone are called "growth lines" (see Fig. 3-38) and reflect a systemic insult at a time when the bone was forming. Determining the normality of the density of bone must take into account the width of the medullary cavity (indicates cortical thickness), the density of the bones generally, and the comparative density of the bone to soft tissue—as an example, the heart as seen on a chest roentgenogram. The determination as to normal, focally abnormal, or totally abnormal density is an important clue in diagnosing bone disease.

Size. The size of an individual bone should be considered in both its length and breadth (Fig. 3-42). The length reflects the ability of the bone to grow at the epiphyseal plates, whereas the width reflects the ability of the bone to respond to stress. The width increases by appositional bone deposit from periosteal attachment. The normal size and habitus as well as hormonal influence determine the usual variations in the thickness and length of the bones. Excess width may result, however, from epiphyseal disturbance producing disordering of the usual modeling of the bone (Fig. 3-43). Hypervascularity following trauma or infec-

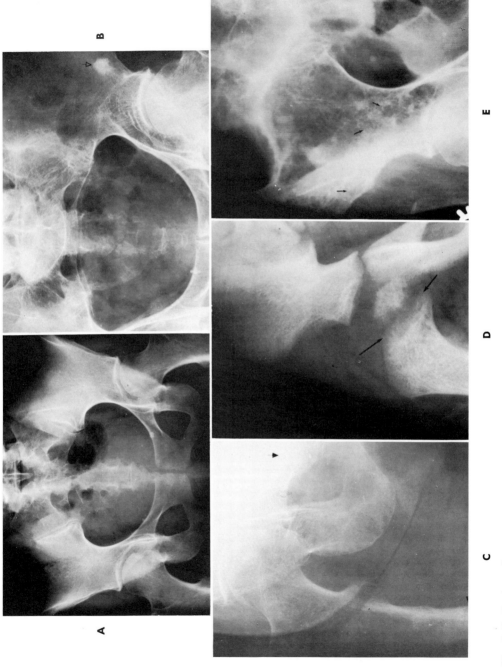

Fig. 3-41. For legend see opposite page.

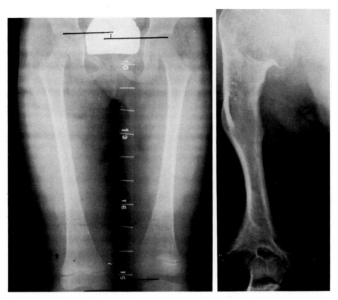

Fig. 3-42   **Fig. 3-43**

Fig. 3-42. Leg length can be measured by roentgenographic techniques utilizing teleoroent-genography with a moving beam. The right leg is a great deal longer than the left; the disparity in length is shown by the distance between the lines indicating the upper and lower ends of the femurs. A rather uneven x-ray tube travel during the time of the exposure causes the irregular transverse densities on the film.

Fig. 3-43. Achondroplasia. This is one of the osseous dystrophies in which the formation of bone at the epiphyseal plate is distorted. The bone is short, broad, and of normal density. This is one of many such dystrophies.

Fig. 3-41. A, Normal appearance of bony pelvis. Notice trabecular pattern and cortical thickness. **B,** Osteoporosis. A prominent trabecular pattern with intact cortices is present. There is an incidental bone island in the left ilium (open arrow). **C,** Osteomalacia. Shows nutritional etiology and generalized demineralization including cortex with pseudofractures (solid arrows). **D,** Osteomalacia in a child with renal rickets shows a broad epiphyseal plate (solid arrows) with diffuse demineralization and poorly defined cortices. **E,** Multiple irregular radiolucencies involve the bony structures of the pelvis (solid arrows). This represents bone replacement by multiple myeloma. The appearance of the bony structures in the other illustrations is that of bony resorption rather than replacement.

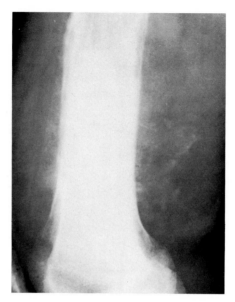

Fig. 3-44. A soft tissue mass about the distal femur, and an increased density of the distal femoral shaft, with linear formation of bony spicules extending into the soft tissues, indicate malignant osteogenic tumor (osteogenic sarcoma in this case).

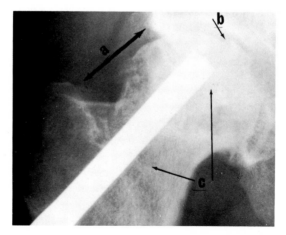

Fig. 3-45. A previous fracture of the femoral neck has been treated by open reduction and placement of a metallic pin through the course of the femoral neck and into the femoral head. The femoral neck is short (double-ended arrow, *a*). A disparate increased density of the femoral head compared to the femoral neck (*c*) is demonstrated. The superior cortical surface (*b*) shows irregular fracturing. The changes of increased density (*c*) and fracturing (*b*), together with the location of the original fracture line, indicate the diagnosis of ischemic necrosis.

tion, or the result of a vascular tumor may produce overgrowth of the length of the bone. Genetic disturbance of mesenchymal differentiation focally or systemically may produce various syndromes or focal gigantism.

Contour. The initial formation of bone and the remodeling of bone produces the final contour. Excess tubulation produces a very thin shaft of the long bone. This may represent poor muscular development secondary to neurologic deficit or various systemic mesenchymal diseases. There may be excess cortical bone in focal areas, which can relate to healing from previous injury or infection. The most common cause for excessive cortical bone deposit is hypertrophic response to aging. This is usually seen at the point of tendinous or ligamentous insertions. Subperiosteal hemorrhage or other causes of periosteal elevation will produce appositional bone and may produce focal irregularity of the contour. A tumor will distort the contour of the bone by focal expansion, by replacement of the bony substance by tumor, or by production of excess bone (Fig. 3-44). Some metabolic disorders, such as acromegaly, predispose to excessive cortical bone, with the contour resembling that observed with degenerative change. The strength of the bone will also affect the final contour since, if the bone is soft, bowing may occur. Abnormal tissue deposited within the medullary cavity can cause widening of portions of the bone, as in, the femora in Gaucher's disease. Abnormalities of maturation of cartilage in the metaphyseal portion may produce widening and irregularities such as seen in achondroplasia.

The major parameters used in determining normality of bone relate to size, density, and configuration, with density and configuration being the major diagnostic clues. Many osseous diseases combine alterations in both of these parameters. Aseptic necrosis, for instance, is manifested by increased density as compared to the adjoining bone. The compression and compaction of the bony substance involved and some resorption of the adjoining bone produce this effect

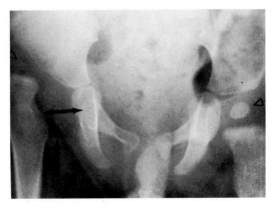

Fig. 3-46. Malalignment (dislocation) is demonstrated. The right femur is displaced laterally from the acetabulum (double-ended broad arrow). The capital femoral epiphysis on the right (open arrow) is quite small compared to that on the left (open arrow). The upward migration of the femur (single arrow) is also shown. The left hip is normal.

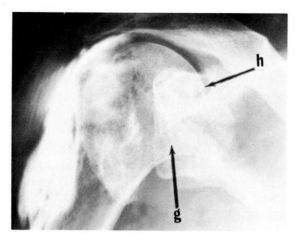

Fig. 3-47. Dislocation of the shoulder may be obscured. The head of the humerus (*h*) lies medial to the articulating surface of the glenoid fossa (*g*). The contrast medium injected into the shoulder joint shows gross distortion along the course of the bicipital tendon, indicating disruption of the tissues.

(Fig. 3-45). Simultaneously, a disturbance of configuration appears due to fragmentation. Differentiation between tumor and infection is difficult and requires careful consideration of variation in density and configuration.

Location. The relative location of one bone to adjoining bones is obviously important in detection of dislocations. Occasionally, in order to fully determine whether there is dislocation at a joint, it will be necessary to have films taken with the x-ray beam at right angles to the other projection. If the margins of the bones comprising the articulations are still cartilaginous, it may be impossible to adequately demonstrate the dislocations roentgenographically. This is particularly true in congenital dislocation of the hip in the infant (Figs. 3-46 and 3-47). The alignment of the appendicular skeleton relative to the torso becomes a diagnostic parameter. "Valgus" and "varus" are terms most commonly used to define the relationship of the lower extremities to the pelvis (Fig. 3-48). They denote the relative alignment of the femoral neck to the acetabulum. If the femoral neck and shaft of the femur form too straight a line, it is considered a valgus ("away from") deformity. In this instance, it is necessary to move the thigh outward laterally from the body in order to produce the normal relationship of the femoral neck and acetabulum. In a varus deformity, the femoral neck and shaft form too acute an angle and requires movement of the femur toward the midline of the body to produce a normal relationship. A similar consideration permits understanding of the term "genu valgus" (knock-knees). The femur must be moved away from the midline of the body to produce the normal tibial femoral alignment. The reverse of this is true with genu varus (bow legs). The adaptive response of the underlying bone to such malalignment can often be seen roentgenographically by altered angle of the articulating surfaces of joints.

Number. Multiple congenital anomalies of the extremities may be manifested

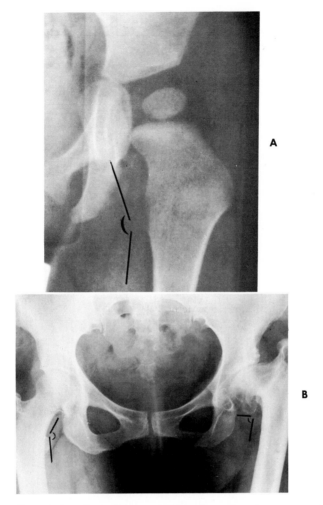

Fig. 3-48. A, Normally a slight valgus alignment of the femoral neck is present in childhood. The lines indicate the angle formed between the femoral neck and the shaft in a normal 2-year-old male. **B,** Varus alignment is manifested by a more acute angle between the femoral neck and shaft of the left hip of this adult. The right hip shows a normal adult alignment.

by either absence of an extremity or absence of one of the bones of an extremity (Fig. 3-49). Certain specific syndromes include aberrations of numbers of toes or fingers and absence of one of the bones of the forearm. The most frequent cause of change in number of appendages, however, is posttraumatic or postsurgical. The absence of the terminal phalanx of one digit may easily be overlooked on a routine roentgenogram.

Margination. The distinctness of outline of the cortex or trabecular pattern is another clue to abnormalities. Loss of sharp cortication is indicative of resorption of calcium or of bone. This may be the result of inflammatory disease of the adjoining soft tissues or of the bone itself. If there is mobilization of the cal-

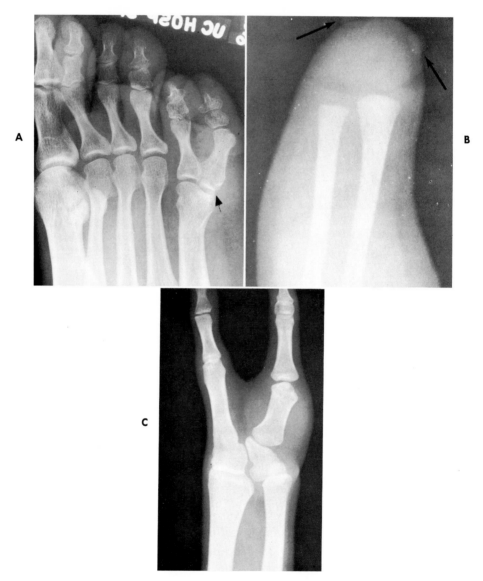

Fig. 3-49. The numbers of digits may vary congenitally. **A,** An accessory small toe (arrow). **B,** Absence of ossifications for the entire hand, with the fingers represented only as small soft tissue buds (arrows). **C,** Congenital failure of the second, third, and fourth digits to develop. There has been fusion of the ossification centers of the carpals so only two are represented; the metacarpal for the ulnar digit is quite broad.

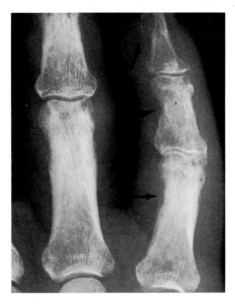

Fig. 3-50. Severe bony resorption may occur as the result of systemic disease, particularly in hyperparathyroidism. The subperiosteal resorption of the midportions of the proximal and middle phalanges and the terminal tuft is indicated by the arrows.

cium stores as the result of metabolic disturbance such as in hyperparathyroidism, subperiosteal cortical resorption occurs as well (Fig. 3-50). A similar effect is produced by elevation of the periosteum by hemorrhage or tumor. Initially, some blurring of the cortical margins occurs. Subsequently lamellar deposits of poorly formed new bone are seen. Irregular resorption of the bone margins around a fracture represents a part of the normal healing process.

REQUIRED READINGS

Caffey, J.: Pediatric x-ray diagnosis, Chicago, 1961, Year Book Medical Publishers, Inc., pp. 747-1156.

Squire, L. F.: Fundamentals of roentgenology, Cambridge, Massachusetts, 1964, Harvard University Press.

RECOMMENDED READINGS

Paul, L. W., and Juhl, J. H.: The essentials of roentgen interpretation, New York, 1964, Harper & Row, Publishers, pp. 3-237.

Pugh, D. G.: Roentgenologic diagnosis of diseases of bones, New York, 1951, Thomas Nelson & Sons.

Weinmann, J. P., and Sicher, H.: Bone and bones, St. Louis, 1950, The C. V. Mosby Co.

ADDITIONAL READINGS

Collins, D. H.: Pathology of bone, London, 1966, Butterworth and Co.

Dahlin, D. C.: Bone tumors, Springfield, Illinois, 1957, Charles C Thomas, Publisher.

Rubin, P.: Dynamic classification of bone dysplasias, Chicago, 1964, Year Book Medical Publishers, Inc.

4

HEAD AND NECK

Summary of basic concepts

  I. Neck
    A. Components
       1. Musculoskeletal
          a. Cervical spine
          b. Angle of mandible
          c. Base of skull
          d. First and second ribs
       2. Respiratory
       3. Digestive
       4. Endocrine
       5. Cardiovascular
       6. Lymphatic
    B. Evaluation of cervical spine
       1. Alignment
          a. Most flexible portion of spine
          b. Usually slightly lordotic but curve determined by position of body and head
          c. Possible abnormalities: scoliosis or kyphosis
       2. Contour (variations from bony overgrowth or loss of bone)
          a. Degenerative disease
          b. Fracture
          c. Long-standing malalignment
          d. Long-standing stress, either compression or tension
       3. Density
          a. Increased (excess bone or calcium)
             (1) Degenerative change
             (2) Healing fracture or infection
             (3) Systemic disease
             (4) Degenerated disc (calcified)
          b. Decreased (loss of bone or calcium)
             (1) Osteoporosis
             (2) Inflammation
             (3) Malignancy
       4. Size
          a. Small vertebrae: focal lack of motion early in life
          b. Size increased: abnormal stress with appositional bone deposit

  c. Abnormally small intervertebral discs
   (1) Degeneration
   (2) Destruction
   (3) Fusion (prolonged lack of motion)
  d. Reduction of posterior structures (laminae, spinous processes, transverse processes)
   (1) Tumor
   (2) Postoperative state
   (3) Development—congenital or lack of motion
 5. Function (indirect evaluation of soft tissues by motion studies)

C. Evaluation of spinal canal
 1. Myelography for study of spinal cord and meninges
 2. Plain film evaluation of bony structures
  a. Pedicles on A-P projection
  b. A-P diameter of canal on lateral projection (posterior margin of vertebral body to anterior aspect of spinous process)
  c. Neural foramina
   (1) Seen in oblique projection
   (2) Part of spinal canal

D. Evaluation of base of skull
 1. Components visible on lateral film of neck
  a. Craniovertebral articulation
  b. Basiocciput
  c. Sella turcica (occasionally)
  d. Atlanto-occipital and atlantoaxial articulations
 2. Parameters
  a. Alignment
   (1) Both on A-P and lateral films: occiput to atlas, odontoid to occiput
   (2) Upward projection of odontoid into foramen magnum with basilar invagination
   (3) Flexion and extension views for stability
  b. Contour
   (1) Normalcy or degenerative changes of apophyseal and craniovertebral joints
   (2) Size of foramen magnum: functional and actual

E. Evaluation of respiratory system
 1. Components
  a. Oropharynx
  b. Hypopharynx
  c. Larynx
  d. Trachea
  e. Vocal cords
  f. Piriform sinuses
 2. Parameters
  a. Density
   (1) Normal
    (a) Air next to soft tissues
    (b) Physiologic calcification cartilages; thyroid, cricoid, arytenoid, tritaceous cartilage
   (2) Abnormal

(a) Calcific or metallic foreign bodies

(b) Calcified lymphoid tissue or tumors

(3) Artificial

(a) Barium for evaluation of oropharynx, hypopharynx

(b) Iodinated substances for larynx and proximal trachea

b. Contour

(1) Irregularity, excess tissues: edema, tumor, infection

(2) Loss of inferior margin true vocal cord: subglottic softtissue mass, either edema or tumor

(3) Reduced size: scarring (destruction, ulceration, postsurgical change), edema, tumor

c. Function

(1) Distensibility or rigidity: tested with fluoroscopy or motion recording

(2) Mobility of vocal cords: tested with fluoroscopy or cineroentgenography with or without laryngogram

(3) Deglutition: rapid action requiring cineroentgenography for complete evaluation

d. Location (in relation to spine and midline)

(1) Midline position of trachea distorted by paratracheal masses

(2) Posterior wall of hypopharynx displaced anteriorly by prevertebral masses

F. Evaluation of endocrine structures

1. Components

a. Thyroid

b. Parathyroid

2. Parameters

a. Density

(1) Usually soft tissue

(2) Not identifiable in normal state

(3) Calcification

(a) Psammous calcification in tumor

(b) Concentric, isolated calcification in adenoma

b. Location

(1) Usually paired structures

(2) Occasionally aberrant glands present

c. Size: increase of component glands

(1) Compression and deviation of trachea

(2) Deviation of esophagus, possibly extending into superior mediastinum

G. Evaluation of digestive system

1. Components

a. Oropharynx   c. Cervical esophagus

b. Hypopharynx   d. Upper portion of thoracic esophagus

2. Parameters

a. Size

(1) Small: scarring, compression, tumor, or edema

(2) Enlarged: obstruction or wall weakness

b. Contour

         (1) Smooth when distended

         (2) Irregularity: tumor, scarring, postsurgical change, foreign bodies

     c. Location

         (1) Displaced: adjoining extrinsic or intrinsic masses

         (2) Retraction: postoperative or postinflammatory scarring

     d. Function: determined by fluoroscopy, cineroentgenography or videotape recording

  H. Evaluation of vascular system

    1. Components (major)

      a. Arterial

         (1) Carotid (common, external, internal)

         (2) Vertebral

         (3) Thyroid and thyrocervical trunk

      b. Venous

         (1) Jugular (internal, external, anterior)

         (2) Perispinal plexus

         (3) Thyroid plexus

         (4) Cervical and vertebral

    2. Parameters

      a. Density

         (1) Naturally occurring—increased: calcification in walls or phleboliths visible

         (2) Artificially induced: venous or arterial injection of iodinated compounds

      b. Size

         (1) Requires opacification to demonstrate

         (2) Lumen may be larger than shown due to streaming or clot or incomplete filling of aneurysm

      c. Location

         (1) Displaced by adjoining masses

         (2) Retracted by postsurgical scarring

      d. Contour

         (1) Tortuosity from degeneration

         (2) Irregularity of lumen from plaque formation

         (3) Sac-like appendage: aneurysm

      e. Number

         (1) Accessory arteries and veins common

         (2) Hypervascularity evident in tumor

         (3) Major vessel not seen if occluded

 I. Evaluation of lymphatic system—parameters

    1. Density

      a. Occasionally calcified following inflammatory disease

      b. Seldom opacified by lymphangiography

    2. Size: enlarged, may displace adjoining structures

II. Skull

  A. Bony envelope of brain, reflecting intrinsic growth potential and adaptation to pressure from within

B. Parameters
  1. Density
     a. Results from inner table, outer table, and diploic structures
     b. Increased density of whole calvarium
        (1) Physiologic
        (2) Total systemic disease
        (3) Diffuse osseous disease
        (4) Reduced intracranial pressure with thick calvarium
     c. Focally increased density
        (1) Physiologic
        (2) Metastatic
        (3) Neoplastic
        (4) Reparative
        (5) Adjoining abnormality
  2. Size
     a. Reflects intracranial pressure
     b. Determined in childhood
  3. Contour
     a. General
        (1) Reflection of pressure and intrinsic potential for bone growth
        (2) Effected by muscular tension
     b. Irregular
        (1) Focal overgrowth
        (2) Unequal pressure
        (3) Muscular imbalance

III. Paranasal sinuses
   A. Components
      1. Frontal
      2. Ethmoid
      3. Maxillary antra
      4. Sphenoid
   B. Parameters
      1. Density (normally air-containing)
         a. Increased density
            (1) Soft tissues or fluid replacing air (amount and configuration of abnormal soft tissue indicative of nature of disease)
            (2) Failure of development—bony
         b. Mucoperiosteal line (lining of sinuses) and density of adjoining bones indicators of normalcy
      2. Size, contour and location
         a. Determining factors
            (1) Communication with air passageway during formative years
            (2) Normalcy of bone around sinuses
            (3) Influence of hormones
         b. Continue to increase in size throughout life
         c. Extensions (normal variants)
            (1) Sphenoids into base of skull

        (2) Ethmoids into supraorbital area

        (3) Antra into hard palate and alveolar ridge of maxilla

    d. Usually asymmetrical

  3. Margination: depends upon aeration, lining of sinuses, adjoining bone

IV. Facial bones and orbits

  A. Parameters

    1. Density

      a. Normal: delicate bones having faint margins

      b. Increased: excess bone formation

        (1) Inflammation

        (2) Tumor

        (3) Metabolic disturbance

      c. Reduced

        (1) Infection

        (2) Osteoporosis

        (3) Tumor

      d. Artificially reduced

        (1) Pneumo-orbitography: air injected behind eyeball to show contents of orbits

      e. Artificially increased

        (1) Arteriography or venography to show vascular structures

      f. Linear radiolucency or increased density in fracture

    2. Size

      a. Factors determining

        (1) Ability of bone to be pneumatized

        (2) Growth potential of bone

        (3) Size of structures contained, such as globe of eye and intraorbital contents

    3. Contour—irregular

      a. Unequal growth of intraorbital structures

      b. Focal variation in growth potential

    4. Location

      a. Hypertelorism: excess distance between orbits

      b. Hypotelorism: reduced distance between orbits

      c. Abnormal location of nasal septum and nasal bone from trauma or developmental variation

    5. Margination

      a. Indicative of status of adjoining structures and bone

      b. Status of adjoining structures by sharpness of outline reflected by superior and inferior orbital fissures, optic foramina, linea innominata

V. Temporal bone

  A. Mastoids

    1. Components

      a. External canal

      b. Facial ridge and canal

      c. Jugular fossa

    d. Stylomastoid foramen

    e. Styloid process

    f. Mastoid air cells

    g. Mastoid antrum

    h. Sinus plate

2. Parameters

    a. Density

        (1) Normally air-containing

        (2) Increased

            (a) Inflammatory disease

                (i) Acute

                (ii) Subacute

                (iii) Chronic and acute

                (iv) Loss of air by fluid formation in subacute

                (v) Loss of air by mucosal thickening and granulation tissue

                (vi) Reparative hyperostosis

            (b) Congenital

                (i) Lack of development of mastoid air cells from early obstructive phenomenon

                (ii) Absence of eustachian tube or tympanic cavity precluding pneumatization

        (3) Reduced: bony destruction

            (a) Tumor

            (b) Cholesteatoma

            (c) Infection

    b. Size

        (1) Marked normal variation

        (2) Dependent upon degree of aeration

        (3) Reduced size reflecting obstruction between nasopharynx and mastoid air cells

        (4) Increased size—a sometimes misleading but normal variant

        (5) Asymmetry most frequent

    c. Contour and margination

        (1) Irregularity of definition effect of abnormality on surrounding tissues

        (2) Loss of mucosal definition from diseased air cells or underlying bone abnormality

    d. Location of air cells

        (1) Usual cellular groups: periantral, lateral, tip cells, zygomatic root, posterior and peritubal, squamosal

        (2) Occasional marked pneumatization of petrous tips

B. Petrous pyramid and middle ear

  1. Components

    a. Internal auditory canal   d. Attic-aditus

    b. Labyrinthine structures   e. Ossicles

    c. Tympanic cavity

  2. Parameters

    a. Density

(1) Normal
    (a) Otic capsule densest cortical bone in body
    (b) Semicircular canals, vestibule and cochlea radiolucent areas within otic capsule
(2) Decreased
    (a) Excessive pneumatization
    (b) Bony destruction
    (c) Osteoporosis
    (d) Enlarged internal auditory meatus and canal
(3) Increased
    (a) Hyperostotic response (reparative)
    (b) Loss of air in middle ear

b. Size
(1) Increased: erosion or normal variant
(2) Decreased: hyperostotic response or failure of development

c. Contour
(1) Middle ear: lens shaped
(2) Internal auditory meatus: juglike contour
(3) Petrous tip: rounded inferior margins

d. Location: ossicular structures displaced by tumor, trauma, or congenital anomaly

e. Reduction in number of ossicles
(1) Destruction
(2) Failure of differentiation

f. Margination
(1) Attic and aditus: evaluate status of adjoining bone in infection or cholesteatoma
(2) Internal auditory meatus: blurred in disease
(3) Lateral margin of lateral semicircular canal: affected by status of mastoid antrum
(4) Sharpness of petrous tip: distorted if invaded by nasopharyngeal tumor

VI. Intracranial structures
  A. Nervous system
    1. Components important to roentgenography
      a. Brain
        (1) Cerebral hemisphere
        (2) Cerebellum
        (3) Septum pellucidum
        (4) Lateral, third, fourth ventricles
        (5) Aquaduct
        (6) Corpus callosum
        (7) Brain stem
        (8) Pineal gland
      b. Pituitary
      c. Meninges
        (1) Pia mater

       (2) Arachnoid

       (3) Dura

    d. Basilar cisterns—subarachnoid

       (1) Cisterna magna

       (2) Chiasmatic cistern

       (3) Pontine cistern

       (4) Interpeduncular cistern

    e. Cranial nerves

2. Parameters

    a. Density

       (1) Normal

          (a) Soft tissue not identifiable on routine films

          (b) Naturally occurring increased calcification

             (i) Pineal (most common)

             (ii) Habenular commissure

             (iii) Choroidal plexus

             (iv) Dura

             (v) Vascular structures (arterial walls)

             (vi) Tumors, abnormalities of vessels

       (2) Artificially reduced

          (a) Air injected via lumbar subarachnoid space and entering ventricles (pneumoencephalogram)

          (b) Air injected into ventricles (ventriculogram)

          (c) Basilar cisterns, subarachnoid spaces and size, configuration, location of ventricular structures depicted

       (3) Artificially increased

          (a) Iodinated substance for visualization of posterior fossa and ventricular system

          (b) Material used similar to that used in myelography

    b. Size

       (1) Reduced in microencephaly

       (2) Increased in hydrocephaly (abnormal tissue)

    c. Contour

       (1) Irregular development of tissue from focal overgrowth or loss of substance

       (2) Structure distortion at some distance from primary abnormality because of compressibility of tissue

    d. Location

       (1) Change by displacement of structures

          (a) Loss of substance on side toward which structures displaced

          (b) Excess tissue on side away from which structure is displaced

       (2) Pineal usually midline, displaced by tumor

       (3) Septum pellucidum altered in location by tumor or mass

    e. Number

       (1) Some basal cisterns paired structures

       (2) If one cistern not seen, indication of abnormality

       (3) Accessory ventricles frequent

B. Vascular structures
   1. Components
      a. Arteries
         (1) Internal carotid
         (2) Anterior cerebral
         (3) Middle cerebral
         (4) Posterior cerebral
         (5) Circle of Willis
         (6) Cerebellar
         (7) Basilar
      b. Veins
         (1) Dural sinuses
         (2) Anastomotic
         (3) Basilar
         (4) Cavernous sinus
         (5) Great vein of Galen
   2. Parameters
      a. Density
         (1) Same density as brain
         (2) Naturally occurring increased: calcification
            (a) Usually related to arteriosclerosis
            (b) May represent abnormalities such as aneurysm or fistula
         (3) Artificially increased
            (a) Induced by intravascular injection through needle or catheter
            (b) Excess contrast in tumor blush
            (c) Reduced contrast in block
            (d) Abnormal channels in anomalies
      b. Size
         (1) Normally variable; tapering as arteries reach periphery and larger as veins reach central collecting areas
         (2) Focal dilatation from aneurysms or excess demand as arteriovenous fistula (may be small in spasm)
      c. Contour
         (1) Normal pattern variable within finite limits
         (2) Loss of normal contour pattern from abnormality of wall
      d. Location
         (1) Predictable in relation to structures of skull
         (2) Displacement from proper location due to loss of substance or excess tissue in areas of brain
         (3) As reliable as evaluation of ventricles of brain in locating certain abnormalities
      e. Number
         (1) Excess in tumors or malformation
         (2) Reduced in spasm or obstruction
         (3) Usually paired structures, except for basilar artery
      f. Margination: sharpness of edge of contrast column lost in aneurysm with clot or extravasation beyond blood vessel, as in hemorrhage or vessel wall rupture

Neck

A cross sectional area of the neck is small compared to one of the torso, but it contains portions of all of the organ systems except the genitourinary tract. Films of the neck demonstrate the musculoskeletal, respiratory (larynx and trachea), digestive (oropharynx, hypopharynx, and cervical esophagus), endocrine (thyroid and parathyroid), vascular (carotid arteries and subjacent branches and jugular veins), lymphatic, and central nervous systems. Naturally occurring densities enable some assessment of most of these systems on a plain film. The air in the trachea, larynx, hypopharynx, and oropharynx, outlines these organs. The laryngeal structures, vocal cords, base of the tongue, epiglottis, portions of the nasopharynx, and occasionally a portion of the cervical esophagus are all outlined (Fig. 4-1). The apices of the lungs may project above the clavicles and be visible on films of the neck. Fat between fascial planes and in the subcutaneous areas is radiolucent and partly delineates lymph nodes in the supra-

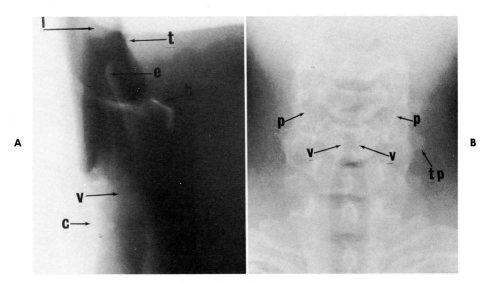

Fig. 4-1. A, The lateral projection of the soft tissues of the cervical area utilizes the contrast of air against soft tissue and calcium within bone to show the normal anatomy. The soft tissue of the tongue (*t*) sets off the anterior margin of the valleculae. The posterior margin is the epiglottis (*e*). These lie superior to the calcification of the hyoid bone (*h*). The cornua of the hyoid extend posteriorly. In the superior portion of the air-filled hypopharynx and oropharynx lies the base of the nasopharynx. The earlobes (*l*) are seen superimposed on the internal structure. They may resemble soft tissue masses in the nasopharynx. Inferiorly, the laryngeal structures show gas between the true and false cords in the laryngeal ventricle (*v*). Calcification in the cricoid cartilages (*c*) identifies the subglottic area. B, In the A-P projection the piriform sinuses (*p*) are identified lying laterally, defined by air. The true cords (*v*) define the entrance to the trachea. The cords are relaxed and there is an air space between them. Immediately below the cord is the subglottic area, which is important in consideration of tumor extension. The transverse processes of the cervical spine (*tp*) can be identified extending laterally.

clavicular regions bilaterally and the margins of the muscle masses. Calcific radiodensity is present in the cervical spine, base of the skull, mandible, and clavicles. Roentgenographic examination of the cervical spine is the most frequent cause for study of this area, although the other organ systems are visible at the same time.

MUSCULOSKELETAL SYSTEM

The components of the musculoskeletal system are; musculature, fascia, ligaments and vertebrae of cervical spine, angle of mandible, base of skull, first and second ribs, and clavicles. Roentgenographic determination of normality of these structures follows that described in the preceding chapter on the osseous system but, certain additional factors are utilized.

Cervical spine

The total and individual alignment of the cervical vertebrae should be studied. This is the most flexible portion of the spine; alterations in alignment have a wide range of normality (Fig. 4-2). Changes in body position or position of the chin relative to the neck affect this alignment. A slight lordosis or anterior curvature of the mid portion of the cervical spine is usually present. As a result a narrow vertical dimension of the posterior part of the intervertebral disc and a high vertical anterior dimension occurs. Loss of the cervical lordosis or a kyphosis (reversed lordosis) may be caused by intrinsic abnormalities of the spine or spasm of the cervical musculature. Scoliosis (lateral curvature) in the cervical spine is fairly common but usually less frequent and less severe than scoliosis in the thoracic region. Usually rotation of one vertebra upon another accompanies the scoliosis. The high degree of flexibility at all levels of the cervical spine allows counter-rotation and straightening of a scoliosis at the craniovertebral junction. While lordosis may reflect muscle spasm, retraction of the chin also produces a lordotic effect. Pathologic reversed lordoses, including muscle spasm, most frequently occur at the C4-5, C5-6 intervertebral disc levels. The predisposition of this part of the spine to reversal of lordosis is to be expected because of the insertions of the anterior cervical musculature. Persistence of reversal of lordosis in extension differentiates between positional malalignment and muscle spasm or other pathologic conditions. Positional reversed lordosis (or kyphosis) vanishes when the neck is extended.

The cervical vertebrae are unique in that uncinate or tonguelike projections are found on the lateral aspect of the vertebral bodies. They are more posteriorly placed in the lower portion of the cervical spine and overlie the intervertebral discs when viewed on roentgenograms. The thinness of the bone prevents easy recognition on lateral projections. The small joints or articular facets lie posterolateral to the vertebral bodies and are placed on the superior and inferior ends of articular pillars or lateral masses. Extending anteriorly and laterally from the articular masses are the transverse processes. The nerve root rests on the transverse process. The vertebral artery penetrates the transverse processes through the foramina transversarium. The pedicles originate fairly high on the vertebral

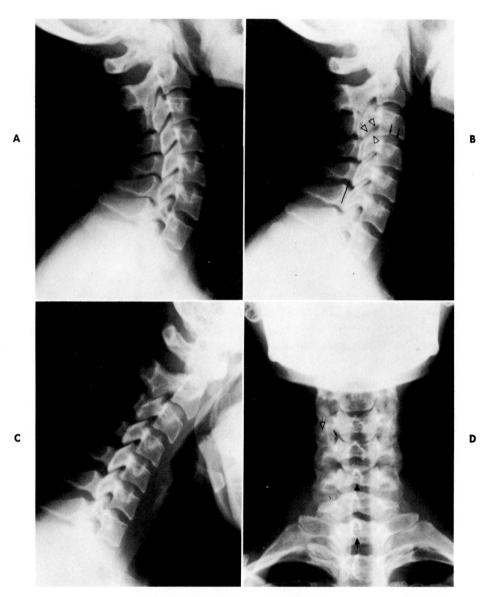

Fig. 4-2. Roentgenographic examination of the cervical spine utilizes the bony density to show the anatomy of the spine and alignment induced by motion to evaluate function. **A,** With the head extended cervical lordosis increases, as compared to the neutral position (**B**). **C,** Cervical lordosis reverses with flexion. Notice the change in form of the intervertebral disc and the variation in alignment of the vertebral bodies with flexion and extension. The migration of the vertebral bodies in a sliding manner is normal if it occurs throughout the cervical spine. The uncinate processes are tongue-like projections from the superior lateral portions of the bodies of the cervical vertebrae (short, solid arrows) and are identifiable in the lateral (**B**) and perhaps better seen in the A-P projection (**D**). They can also be identified in the oblique projection (**E**). They overlie the intervertebral disc. The spinous processes (broad, solid arrows) are visible in the lateral projection (**B**) extending posteriorly and in the A-P projection (**D**—round white rings).

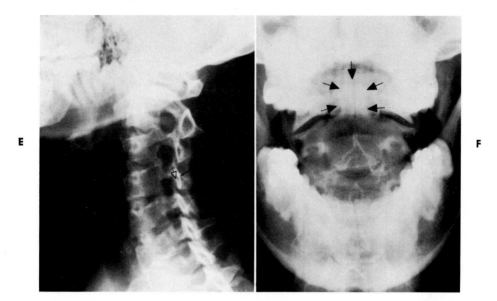

Fig. 4-2, cont'd. E, The laminae, which extend from the base of the spinous processes to the articulating masses posteriorly (long thin arrows), are most easily identified on the oblique projections as white teardrops. The apophysial articulations or posterior small joints (open arrows) can be seen in the lateral, oblique, and A-P projections. The odontoid is observed in both the lateral and the special A-P projection (**F**), which is done with the mouth open.

bodies and comprise the roof and floor of the neural foramina. The nerve roots, therefore, are surrounded by bone originating from ossification centers which first appear posteriorly. An oblique position of the cervical spine is necessary for roentgenographic demonstration of the neural foramina, which angle outward and anteriorly at approximately 45° from the spinal canal. Reduction in the cross sectional area of the neural foramina frequently occurs with aging, as a result of excessive bone deposit in the form of hypertrophic spurs or fringing on the uncinate processes. If the transverse processes are long, they can be identified on the lateral film of the cervical spine, extending beyond the anterior margin of the vertebral body. The unique mobility of the cervical spine accentuates the lesser anterior-posterior dimension of the superior margin of the vertebral body compared to the inferior margin. The overriding of one vertebral body on another in flexion adds to this discrepancy.

Long-standing malalignment produces adaptive changes in the contour of the vertebrae in all areas of the spine. Thus, a discrepancy in leg length produces a tilt of the pelvis and concomitant scoliosis in the lumbar and thoracic area and frequently in the cervical area as well. Bone of a vertebral body growing under compression becomes more dense but develops less vertical dimension. A vertebral body growing under relative tension has increased vertical dimension but less degree of density. While fractures of the cervical spine are not rare, the normal contour is so variable because of the stress of mobility that detection of minor compression fractures is difficult. In addition, delicateness of the bony structure and the complexity of the individual vertebrae make detection of minor linear fractures almost impossible. It may be necessary to obtain follow-up films after the bone has repaired in order to substantiate that a fracture once existed.

The cervical vertebral bodies are small and the laminae are quite thin making demineralization difficult to demonstrate. The overlying transverse processes produce apparent irregular areas of increased or focal areas of decreased density of the vertebral bodies when seen on the lateral projections. Increased density along the margins of the uncinate processes and the adjoining area of the vertebral bodies, caused by hypertrophic degenerative change, may appear on the lateral projection as a relatively radiolucent line transversing the vertebral body. This is easily mistaken for a fracture. An example of such a line is shown in Fig. 4-3. Systemic disease such as osteosclerosis or metastasis, healing fracture, infection, and hypertrophic bony response to degenerative change are all causes of increased radiodensity. Osteoporosis, metastasis, and inflammation account for decreased density in approximately that order. Calcifications may occur in the intervertebral discs from degeneration of aging or fixation of adjoining vertebrae. The disc then is denser and narrower in its vertical dimension than the normal disc.

Vertebral size is highly variable. Fixation of vertebrae at an early age produces small anteroposterior diameters of the vertebral bodies (Fig. 4-4). General musculoskeletal development and sex also determine in part the size of the individual structures. Abnormal stress may increase the vertebral size as the result of appositional bone deposit.

Normal variation occurs in the size of the intervertebral discs. Usually the vertical dimension progressively increases from the upper to the lower cervical spine segments until the level of the C6-7 disc, which may normally be smaller than the C5-6 disc. Degeneration, destruction due to infection, trauma, lack of motion due to fusion, or relative fixation contributes to loss of substance of the intervertebral disc.

The posterior structures of the vertebrae (laminae, spinous processes, and transverse processes) show extensive variation in size. Change in size of these structures may result from tumor, postoperative state, developmental aberrations, or racial variation.

The cross sectional area of the vertebrae in the cervical region compared to the total muscle mass is extremely small. The cervical spine can be thought of as the flexible center pole of a circus tent responsive to stress from the supporting guy wires of the ligaments and muscles. Due to the complexity of the musculature, it is difficult to evaluate the soft tissues directly on routine roentgenograms. Functional studies using cineroentgenography or flexion, extension, and rotation films allow indirect assessment of the normality of the soft tissues.

The spinal cord is nonradiopaque and is only indirectly assessed on the routine film study. The size of the bony spinal canal is shown by the distance between the pedicles, seen on an A-P projection of the cervical spine, and the distance between the base of the spinous process and the posterior surface of

Text continued on p. 200.

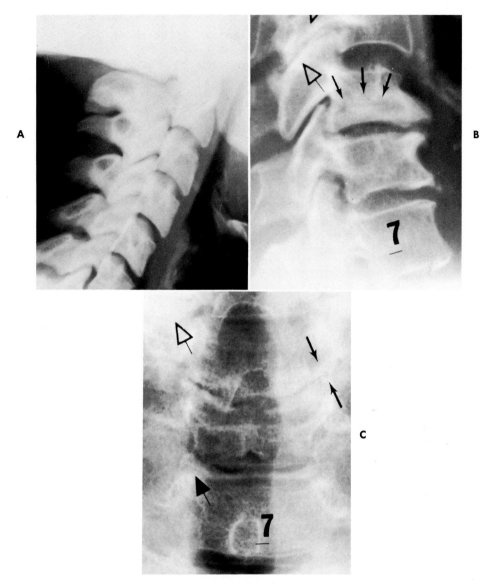

Fig. 4-3. Variations in form and density in the cervical spine are clues to disease. **A,** The osseous structures as a whole are abnormally dense as the result of abnormal conversion of osteoid to bone with excess calcification (osteopetrosis). **B** and **C,** In contrast, focal increased density and bony overgrowth are common findings in degenerative change. Spur formation occurs on the anterior aspect of the vertebral bodies from degeneration and around the apophysial joints (open arrows). In **B** a radiolucent line (small arrows) crosses the body of the fifth cervical vertebra. In **C** this line is shown to be the overgrowth about the appositional area of the uncinate process of the sixth cervical vertebra and the adjoining margin of the body of the fifth cervical vertebra (small arrows). A more normal uncinate process (broad solid arrow) is seen on the seventh cervical vertebra. The overgrowth about the apophysial joints is again observed (open arrows).

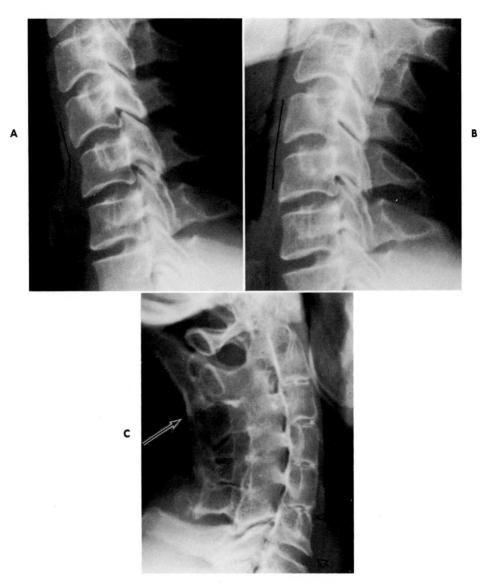

Fig. 4-4. Alignment as affected by motion, size, and form provides clues to normality. There is a reversal of the usual lordosis (**A**) in the neutral position; it corrects fairly well in extension (**B**), as demonstrated by the angles shown by the solid lines. This may result from muscle spasm, but the degree of correction of the reversed lordosis in extension indicates that this is not a major anatomic derangement. In contrast, posterior fusion at an early age (**C**) produces a change in the form of the vertebral body (open arrows) between the areas where motion is present and not present. The A-P diameter of the vertebral bodies increases where motion occurs. The intervertebral disc between the nonmobile segments becomes small and calcified, and the anterior posterior dimension of the vertebral bodies remains decreased. The major anteroposterior growth of the vertebral bodies depends upon appositional bone formation anteriorly caused by motion. The solid posterior bony mass as the result of fusion (broad arrow) can be identified.

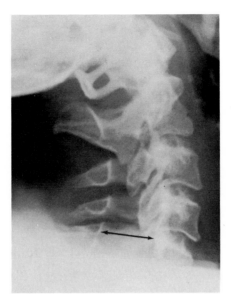

Fig. 4-5. Change in the diameter of the spinal canal (double-ended arrow) results from increased pressure within the canal. The common.cause for this is a longstanding tumor. In this instance, however, it is the result of tuberculosis of the high thoracic spine producing a hunchback configuration of the spine.

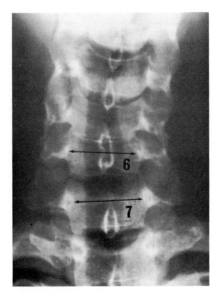

Fig. 4-6. In the A-P view of the cervical spine the distance between the pedicles (double-ended arrows) is a gauge of the size of the contents of the canal. The pedicles of the sixth cervical vertebra have been flattened and eroded by a tumor lying within the spinal cord. The appearance of the pedicles of the seventh cervical vertebra is normal. The white teardrop-shaped densities lying along the course of the spinal canal represent the spinous processes.

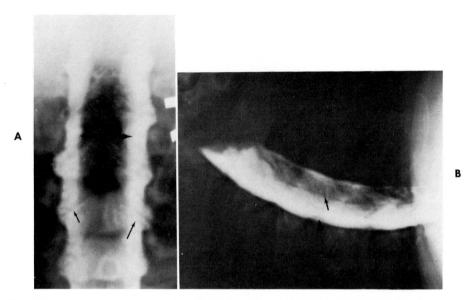

Fig. 4-7. A, Introduction of an oily iodinated medium into the spinal canal (myelography) makes the outline of the spinal cord (double-ended arrow) visible. The nerve rootlets (small arrows) can also be identified as they leave the cord and pass through the axillary pouches of the arachnoid and dura. This is a normal appearance. **B,** The lateral projection, taken at the same time as **A** with the patient in the prone position, shows the small nerve rootlets (small arrow) coming from the posterior aspect of the cord toward the nerve root pouch. A small impression on the anterior aspect of the contrast medium (large arrow) indicates the bulge of a herniated nucleus pulposus. **C,** In contrast to the normal width of the spinal cord as seen in **A,** diffuse enlargement of the spinal cord by a fluid-filled mass (**C,** double-ended arrow) narrows the lateral collection of contrast medium (apposing arrows). **D,** During myelography the contrast medium may be passed through the foramen magnum into the lower portion of the posterior fossa. The impression on the anterior aspect of the contrast column by the odontoid (open arrow) produces a rounded radiolucency. Just superior (small arrow) is the outline of the anterior spinal artery. Immediately above that the vertebral arteries entering the posterior fossa through the anterior aspect of the foramen magnum (lower solid arrows) course toward the midline to form the basilar artery (apposing solid arrows). If the head is elevated, the contrast medium will easily flow back out of the posterior fossa. The *R* lying at the bottom of the film with a small droplet in the center is a mercury marker with the droplet of mercury indicating the direction of tilt of the patient. The marker indicates that the head is lower than the feet. **E, F,** Introduction of iodinated compound directly into the nucleus pulposus (discography) demonstrates the internal structure of the disc. The small arrows indicate the posterior extension of the contrast medium, with the needles entering the discs through the anterior soft tissues of the neck on the right side. The extension of the contrast medium indicates that there is rupture of the annulus fibrosis. The lateral projection (**E**) also shows that an anterior interbody fusion has been accomplished between the bodies of the fifth and sixth cervical vertebrae. This is one surgical treatment for degenerative disc disease. In the A-P projection (**F**) it is seen that the contrast medium escapes laterally as well as posteriorly (thin long arrows). It then reaches to the level of the neural foramina which lie at the tip of the arrows.

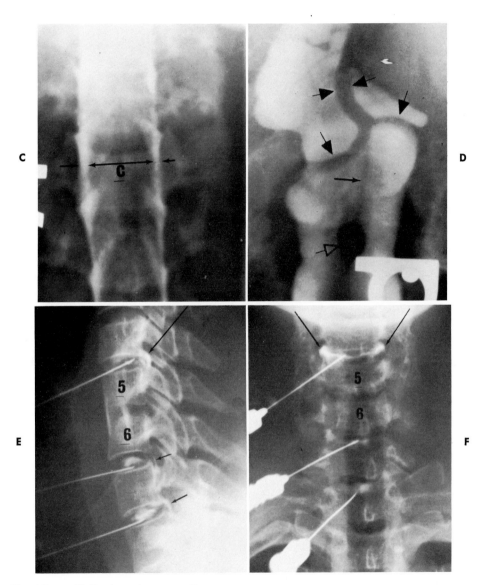

Fig. 4-7, cont'd. For legend see opposite page.

the vertebral bodies (Figs. 4-5 and 4-6). Charts showing the normal measurements of these diameters are available. Myelography is necessary for more complete study of the spinal canal and spinal cord. A positive contrast medium is usually used, but in the high cervical segments and the region of the foramen magnum, air myelography gives more complete information. The neural foramina are actually part of the spinal canal, and the meninges continue along the course of the nerve roots into the neural foramina (Fig. 4-7).

Base of skull

The lateral films of the neck or cervical spine provide an excellent view of the base of the skull and the craniovertebral articulation. Usually lateral projection films of the cervical spine are obtained without rotation of the head on the neck, giving an accurate depiction of the high cervical structures. The basiocciput and base of the skull can usually be seen almost to the region of the sella turcica.

The atlanto-occipital and atlantoaxial articulations

The atlas can be thought of as a washer interposed between the base of the skull and the spine, allowing a high degree of rotation and some flexion and extension.

Alignment. The orientation of the base of the skull and the atlas should be reviewed in both the A-P and lateral projections to detect any malalignment at the atlanto-occipital junction. The atlas tends to follow the skull in motion, so

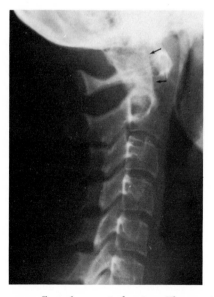

Fig. 4-8. Systemic disease may affect the cervical spine. The erosion of the anterior aspect of the odontoid (small arrows) and the separation of the anterior arch of the atlas from the odontoid indicate effusion. Both of these changes are the result of rheumatoid arthritis.

that the C1-C2 relationship is more frequently disturbed. The tip of the odontoid or dens, should lie at or below the edge of the foramen magnum. Invagination of the base of the skull or congenital abnormalities of the cranioverterbral articulation may allow the odontoid to lie too high. This causes narrowing of the foramen magnum. Muscle spasm (torticollis) or diseases weakening the atlantooccipital membrane may cause counterrotation of the skull on the atlas or on the axis (Fig. 4-8). Flexion and extension views in the lateral projection will determine the degree of stability between C1 and C2.

Density. Focally decreased density of the odontoid and the anterior arch of the atlas results from inflammatory disease of the articulations between these two osseous structures. Rheumatoid arthritis and inflammatory disease of the nasopharynx in childhood are two examples. The lymphatics draining the nasopharynx and the oropharynx anastomose with lymphatics from this articulation. It is possible for infection to involve this joint from the pharyngeal area.

Contour. The vertebral arteries pass through the foramina transversarium, of C1, swing posteriorly, and enter the skull through the foramen magnum. A notch is produced on the posterior lateral aspect of the atlas along the course of these arteries. The joints between C1 and C2 and C1 and the base of the skull may show distortion from the hypertrophic response of degeneration. The margins of the foramen magnum are seen anteriorly at the tip of the basiocciput and posteriorly at the junction of the inner table and the outer table of the occipital bone. This distance is the actual size of the foramen magnum. The functional size depends upon the relation of the odontoid to the foramen magnum.

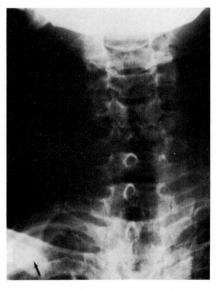

Fig. 4-9. The upper portion of the thoracic cage is seen on the roentgenograms of the cervical spine. Destruction of the right third rib (solid arrow) is the result of invasion by bronchogenic carcinoma.

If the odontoid projects into the foramen magnum, sufficient narrowing may occur to produce neurologic deficit.

Portions of the mandible and the temporomandibular articulation are occasionally demonstrated on films of the neck. The attitude of the head is shown by the relationship of the mandible to the cervical spine. A flexed attitude of the head produces a reversed lordosis of the midcervical spine.

The posterior parts of the first and second ribs and the upper portion of the clavicles are seen on A-P films of the cervical spine. Overdevelopment of the costal elements of the seventh cervical vertebra (cervical rib) can be shown by this method. Normally, the transverse processes of C7 in the adult are shorter than those of T1. The reverse proportion is found in childhood. Destructive processes of the posterior aspect of the first and second ribs may best be demonstrated on films of the cervical spine (Fig. 4-9).

RESPIRATORY SYSTEM

Density. The air within the lumen of the structures of the respiratory system makes it possible to see them. Calcific densities do occur in the laryngeal cartilages and may provide confusing overlapping shadows. The tritaceous cartilage lies posterior to the air within the hypopharyngeal structures and may be mistaken for an opaque foreign body (Fig. 4-10). On occasion, calcific or metallic foreign bodies are lodged in the respiratory tract in the cervical area and are demonstrated on roentgenograms. Fish and fowl bones are thin structures frequently suspected as foreign bodies. Careful technique is required to demonstrate them.

More definitive studies require artificially induced contrast. Barium sulfate is most widely used for evaluation of the oropharynx and hypopharynx (Fig. 4-11). Demonstration of the laryngeal structures and the cervical portion of the trachea is accomplished using iodinated oily media (laryngography). Good coating of the mucosa provides excellent definition of the intrinsic structures.

Contour. Knowledge of the normal appearance of the respiratory structures in the cervical area is required to utilize roentgenograms of this area. The prominence of the false cords immediately above and the true cords immediately beneath the laryngeal ventricle and the subglottic area are well shown on a proper A-P view of the neck. Excess tissue in the subglottic region may represent edema or invasion by tumor. The margination of the cords may be impaired by tumor. The laryngeal vestibule and the pyriform sinuses should show a configuration comparable to that illustrated in Fig. 4-12. Reduction in the size of the cavities and irregularity of contour reflects distortion of the soft tissues as by scarring, destruction by tumor or trauma, ulceration, postsurgical effect, or edema.

Function. Roentgenographic study of the motion of the hypopharyngeal and laryngeal components provides information about the status of these tissues. Cineroentgenographs (x-ray movies) are now being used to demonstrate the distensibility of the pyriform sinuses and the mobility of the vocal cords. Carefully performed fluoroscopy is also a satisfactory method of studying these structures. It is less adequate than cineroentgenographs because the act of swallowing is an ex-

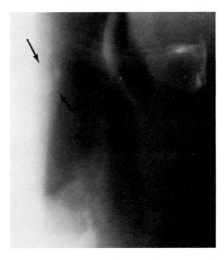

Fig. 4-10. The cartilago triticea is a small cartilage lying in the thyrohyoid membrane. This may calcify. In this case, confusion resulted because the patient gave a history of discomfort in the hypopharynx since having eaten chicken. The arrows point to the calcification which was initially mistaken as an osseous foreign body.

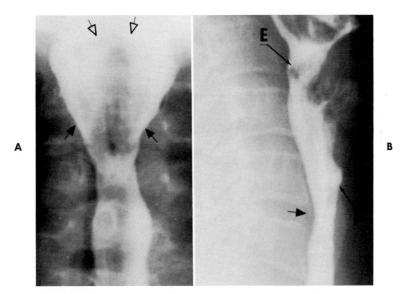

Fig. 4-11. A, The ingestion of barium defines the margins of the hypopharynx and cervical esophagus. The epiglottis (open arrows) covers the entrance to the laryngeal vestibule during swallowing, with distention of the piriform sinuses (solid arrows); the barium spills over into the cervical esophagus. This is a normal appearance seen during the act of swallowing. **B,** Lateral vew of the hypopharyngeal esophageal area outlined with barium shows the same anatomic structures as seen in A-P projection (**A**). The epiglottis (*E*) is observed to be folded over the laryngeal vestibule. The piriform sinuses (*P*) project somewhat anteriorly. The barium passes into the cervical esophagus from the piriform sinuses with some anterior position of the esophagus (solid arrow) over a minor anterior bulge of the intervertebral disc. This is a normal appearance.

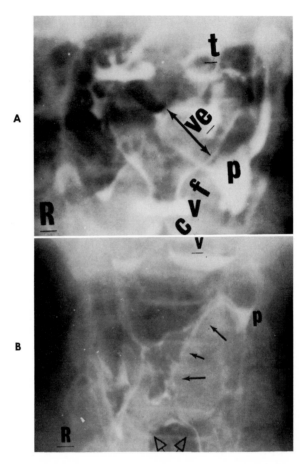

Fig. 4-12. A, It is possible to increase the density of the soft tissues of the larynx by introducing an iodinated compound. The general structures of this larynx are normal with the contrast medium having first opacified the valleculae. The left vallecula is distorted by a small tumor mass (*t*). The contrast medium then outlines the laryngeal ventricle (*ve*), with the double-ended arrow pointing to the level of the incisura of the posterior margin of the vestibule. The posterior wall of the vestibule is the aryepiglottic fold. The contrast medium then passes over the false cord (*f*) to define the laryngeal ventricle (*v*), which separates the false from the true cords (*c*). Below the true cords is the subglottic space. The piriform sinuses are identifiable on either side (*p*). **B,** The distortion of the laryngeal structures by disease contrasts with the appearance seen in **A.** The left vallecula (*v*) is broad and shallow and the left piriform sinus (*p*) is short and elevated. Soft tissue, representing tumor and edema, is contrasted against the iodinated compound and air in the laryngeal vestibule (small, solid arrows). The subglottic space (open arrows) is normal. The artificial change in density added to normal contrast between air and soft tissue makes identification of the abnormality possible.

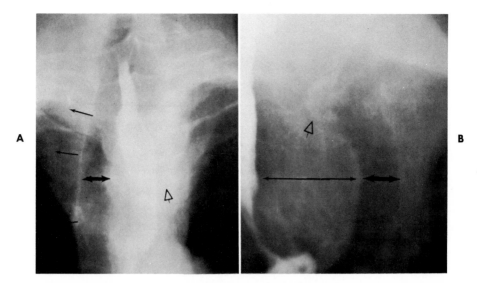

Fig. 4-13. A, Distortion of the location and form of normal structures together with naturally occurring and artificially induced changes in density are illustrated. A soft tissue mass lies behind the manubrium, causing tracheal deviation to the right and some narrowing of the trachea (short, broad, double-ended arrow). Some densities are observed within the mass itself (open arrow). The tracheal shift to the right (small solid arrows) indicates that the mass lies in the left suprasternal notch area and retrosternal area. **B,** When viewed in the lateral projection the mass extends inferiorly to lie between the trachea (double arrow) and the esophagus producing an increased space (long thin arrow). The calcific densities within the mass (open arrow) identify the location. This represents a massive enlargement of the thyroid extending into the mediastinum with calcification indicating adenoma formation.

tremely rapid series of muscular actions in the posterior oropharynx and hypopharyngeal area. These structures change in form and location during swallowing. The epiglottis, hyoid bone, larynx, and pyriform sinuses are usually in motion at the same time.

Location. The trachea normally lies in the midline; however, adjoining excess soft tissue may displace the trachea. Unilateral enlargement of the thyroid is a common cause of such a shift. Scarring of the soft tissues or displacement by inflammatory or tumor masses also causes tracheal deviation (Fig. 4-13). Prevertebral masses, such as abscess or tumor, may displace the posterior wall of the hypopharynx. Muscle spasm of the anterior cervical musculature causes an apparent hypopharyngeal displacement.

DIGESTIVE SYSTEM

The oropharynx and hypopharynx provide a common channel for the digestive and respiratory systems. The digestive tract (esophagus) in this area is of soft tissue density. Artificially induced contrast is required to delineate the details of the structures. The size of the structures depends upon the degree of distention. A small lumen may result from scarring, tumor, or compression (Fig. 4-14). Obstruction to the passage of food or fluids in the esophagus causes dila-

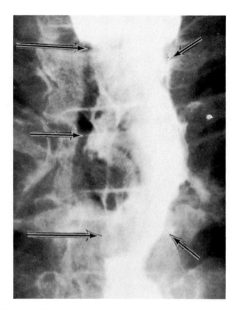

Fig. 4-14. Distortion of form and irregularity of the low cervical esophagus outlined by barium. There are multiple irregularities of the wall (arrows) and the lumen is abnormal. Since all the walls of the esophagus are involved, this represents a encircling lesion. This is a carcinoma of the esophagus.

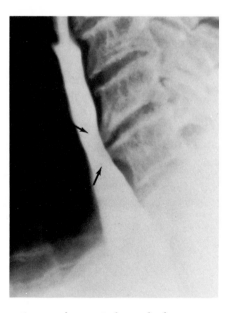

Fig. 4-15. Bony spur formation on the cervical vertebral may encroach on the barium filled esophagus and potentially interfere with swallowing. A crescentic decreased density within the central portion of the barium filled esophagus (arrow) shows the extent of the deformity. The esophagus is displaced slightly to one side.

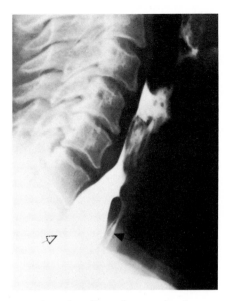

Fig. 4-16. Occasionally the esophageal wall weakens and a large sac or diverticulum forms. The collection of barium in the blind pocket (open arrow) lies behind the lower cervical esophagus (solid arrow). The diverticula, when large, may cause some obstruction and difficulty in swallowing.

tation of the more proximal portion of the esophagus. Functional roentgenographic recording provides the best evaluation of size, since peristalsis produces a continuous change in esophageal diameter.

Contour. The components of the digestive system in the cervical area show smooth margins when distended. Loss of normal tissue of the wall or lining or tumor masses projecting into the lumen cause abnormality of the contour.

Location. The pyriform sinuses normally lie lateral and somewhat posterior to the laryngeal vestibule. The aryepiglottic folds and epiglottis provide a sloping anterior wall to this portion of the hypopharynx. The cervical esophagus lies in close apposition to the anterior aspect of the vertebral bodies of the cervical spine. Distortion of contour of the esophagus is seen if anterior spurs have developed on the vertebral bodies (Fig. 4-15). The esophagus is easily displaced by adjoining masses, either intrinsic or extrinsic. Retraction can result from scarring, postoperative state, or postinflammatory changes. An esophageal diverticulum (Zenker's diverticulum) can distort the contour and location of the esophagus in the cervical area (Fig. 4-16). The esophagus normally describes an arc to the left in the suprasternal notch area, but the sweep can be accentuated by adjoining structures.

ENDOCRINE SYSTEM

The thyroid and parathyroid glands lie in the cervical region. These glands are normally of soft tissue density and therefore not identifiable unless they distort surrounding tissue. If the thyroid is big enough it can be seen as a soft tissue prominence anterior to the trachea on a lateral projection of the neck. Distortion of the trachea and the subcutaneous fat may ensue. Tracheal and esophageal deviation to either side can be seen on routine films with barium outlining the esophagus. Parathyroid adenomas do not usually produce plain film aberrations but require barium studies of the esophagus to demonstrate their presence. Calcification is occasionally detected (see Fig. 4-13). The type of calcification may define the type of tissue present. Psammous calcifications occur in tumors of the thyroid, whereas concentric isolated calcifications occur in thyroid adenomas. The thyroid may enlarge sufficiently to extend into the retromanubrial or retrosternal area of the superior mediastinum.

VASCULAR SYSTEM

Opacification of the vascular structures by injection of iodinated compounds has given rise to a whole field of diagnostic study. The reader is referred to definitive works on this subject for detailed description of the anatomy and its variations and abnormalities. The normal density of the arteries and veins is the same as that of the adjoining soft tissues and cannot be identified on plain films. Calcium deposits in the walls of the arteries can be seen. Occasionally, calcification within an arterial wall is mistaken for a radiopaque foreign body in the esophagus on lateral films of the neck. The size of the vessels is shown only by opacification studies and even this method may not depict the total size of the lumen. Streaming or layering of the contrast medium along the dependent portion of the lumen of the vessel may cause the size to appear smaller than it really is. Enlarged tortuous vessels may result from degeneration of the arterial wall and may displace adjoining structures, such as the trachea. The use of con-

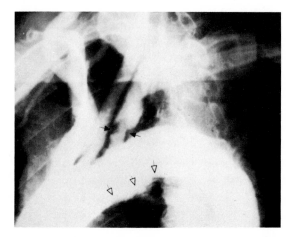

Fig. 4-17. By changing the contrast within the arterial tree by injection of an iodinated compound arterial abnormalities can be shown. In contrast to the normal study, the wall of the aorta (open arrows) is grossly irregular as the result of atheromatous disease. The size of the left subclavian artery (solid arrows) has been sharply reduced by similar disease process.

trast medium permits delineation of accessory vessels, hypervascularity of tumors, aneurysmal dilatation of vessels, irregularity of lumen from arteriosclerotic plaque formation, and blocking of the vessels by clot (Fig. 4-17).

LYMPHATIC SYSTEM

Extensive lymph channels and lymph nodes are present in the cervical area. These normally are not identifiable roentgenographically unless there is rather marked enlargement. If this occurs, displacement or irregularity of the outlines of the subcutaneous fat and the supraclavicular fat pads results (Fig. 4-18). Lymphangiography (injections of iodinated compounds into the soft tissues of the feet) may show opacification of some of the left supraclavicular nodes. The lymph nodes calcify as the result of scarring from previous inflammatory disease

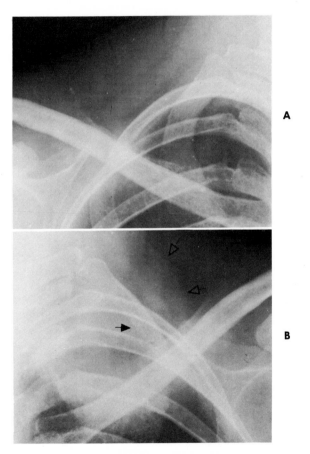

Fig. 4-18. Utilizing the normal roentgenographic densities in the supraclavicular area, certain disease processes or abnormalities can be detected. **A,** In the normal supraclavicular area the supraclavicular fat pad is identified as a radiolucent triangle lying above the clavicle and lateral to the ribs, with the muscle bundles seen passing through this region. **B,** A mass distorts the form of the fat pad (open arrows). This case represents a carcinoma of the lung which has extended into the supraclavicular area. Notice that the first rib has been eroded (solid arrow).

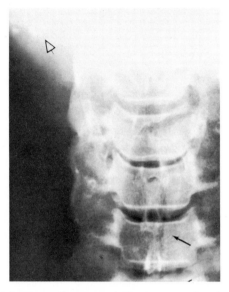

Fig. 4-19. Occasionally infection will cause calcification in nodes (open arrow) which must be identified. This patient also shows some deviation of the trachea (solid arrows) by an enlarged thyroid.

and are discernible on plain films (Fig. 4-19). These calcific deposits may be confused with arterial calcifications or radiopaque intraluminal foreign bodies in the respiratory or digestive tract. Distortion of the soft tissues results from radical surgical removal of the lymph nodes and is seen on the roentgenographs.

Head

SKULL

The form of the skull is a product of intrinsic growth potential and adaptation to pressure from the growing brain. Capacity for growth depends on the cranial sutures (Figs. 4-20 to 4-24).

Density. The normal density of the skull is dependent upon age, sex, hormonal state, variation in vascularity, and individual characteristics. There is a normal variation in the radiodensity of different areas of the skull. The bone about the suture margins contains very little diploë and remains increased in density throughout life. Radiodensity of the skull comes from superimposed outer table, inner table, and the diploic structures. Variation in the calcium content or thickness of any of these layers affects the radiographic density. It is important to determine whether any change in radiodensity reflects alteration in the outer table, inner table, or the diploic space. Varying disease processes affect each of these individual areas (Fig. 4-25).

The skull as a whole may be increased in density. A systemic disease should

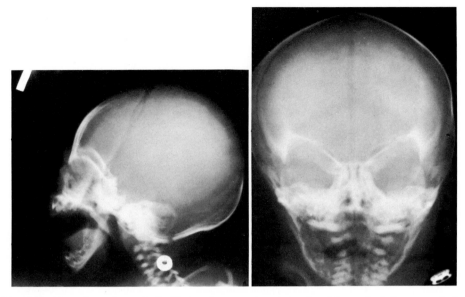

Fig. 4-20. Normal newborn skull. Notice the patent sutures, the thin parietal bones, and the relative size of the cranial vault as compared to the facial bones.

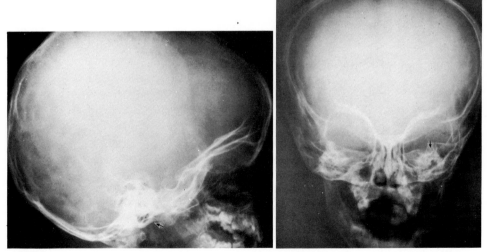

Fig. 4-21. Normal 14-month-old child. The sutures are closing but the lambdoidal, coronal, and sagittal sutures are still patent. Aeration is developing in the mastoids and maxillary antra. **A,** On the lateral projection the ossification center for the bony portion of the external auditory canal is seen to extend well below the base of the skull (solid arrow). **B,** The structures of the labyrinth of the middle ear (solid arrow) are well seen on the A-P projection.

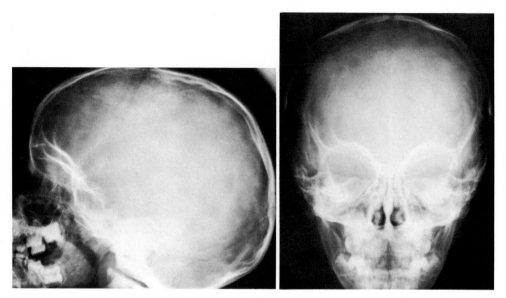

Fig. 4-22. Normal two-year-old child's skull. Closure of the sutures has progressed but the anterior fontanel is still patent. Notice the relative change in the cranial vault size compared to the facial bone size. This is beginning to approximate adult ratio.

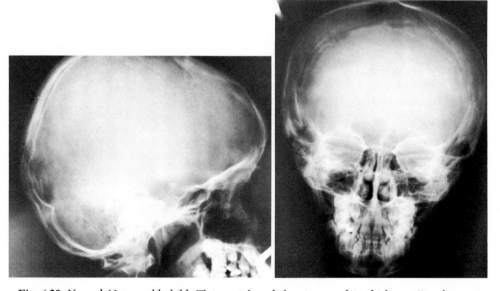

Fig. 4-23. Normal 11-year-old child. The cranial vault has increased in thickness. Development of the frontal sinuses has occurred, and there has been progressive pneumatization of the mastoids.

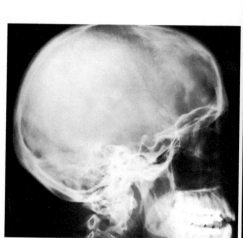
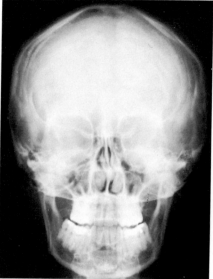

Fig. 4-24. Normal adult skull. Some normal sclerosis and minor irregular radioluency are evident along the course of the closed sutures. The mastoid air cells and the paranasal sinuses are now completely developed.

be suspected with the skull being only a part of the total skeletal osteosclerosis. A thin diploë with heavy inner and outer tables produces a relatively increased physiologic density. The thickness and density of the skull may be accentuated in individuals who have had diseases increasing the function of the bone marrow of the diploic space. Underdevelopment of the brain produces a thick inner table and general increase in density (Fig. 4-26).

The increased density may be focal. The frontal bone frequently develops a physiologic hyperostosis of the inner table in the adult. Metastatic disease, primary neoplastic disease, reparative change from trauma or infection, or response to adjoining soft tissue abnormality, such as infection, all are causes of focal increase in density.

Size. The final size of the skull is determined by intracranial pressure and potential for development (Figs. 4-27 and 4-28). Early fusion of the cranial sutures prevents the effect of the growth of the brain on the skull size.

Contour. The effect of the growing brain, muscular pull from the cervical musculature, abnormal weight-bearing alignment as from scoliosis or kyphosis, or softening of the calvarium by inadequate bone formation can all produce irregularities of the skull contour. Focal irregularity of contours results if one area of the skull loses its potential for growth. A focal area of the skull may have excess potential for growth (benign osteoma) producing irregularity. Certain diseases, such as Paget's disease, produce irregularity of the skull, thickening of the diploë and apparent cranial enlargement in adulthood. Generally, the form and size of the skull are determined by adolescence (See Fig. 4-25).

A   B

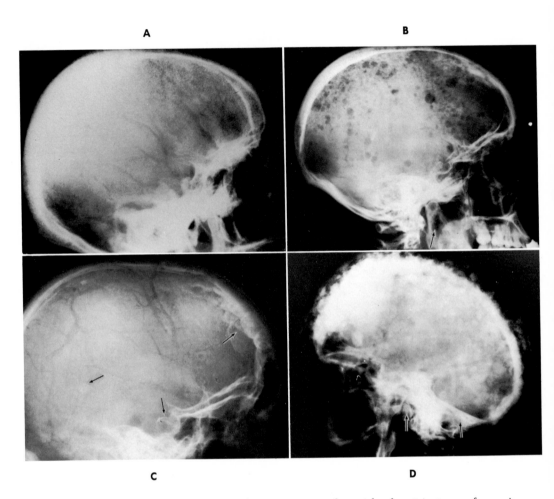

C   D

Fig. 4-25. **A,** Increased activity of the bone marrow as the result of certain types of anemia produces new bone formation which resembles hair on end. Sickle cell anemia is illustrated here. **B,** Multiple myeloma produces punched out multiple radiolucent areas scattered throughout the skull. The mandible is also involved (arrow). **C,** Density may be increased. Hyperostosis frontalis interna (open arrow) is a common physiologic thickening of the inner table of the calvarium corresponding to the convolutions of the brain. The solid arrow indicates calcification of the diaphragma sellae; the linear calcification below that is the internal carotid artery. Posteriorly, a large calcific deposit lies in the region of the choroidal plexuses (broad solid arrow). **D,** Irregular hyperostosis and lucency is the characteristic appearance of Paget's disease, a disease of unknown etiology affecting older individuals. There is softening of the bone as evidenced by some intrusion of the cervical spine into the base of the skull (solid arrows).

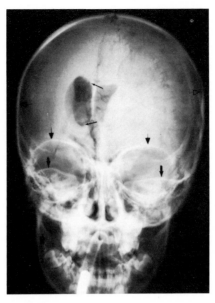

Fig. 4-26. The size and form of the cranial structures may be altered. There is unilateral cerebral atrophy with the calvarium on the right being thicker than that on the left (open arrows). The petrous ridge and orbital roof on the right lie higher than on the left (broad, solid arrows). The lateral ventricle on the right is enlarged as compared to the left, and there is some migration toward the right (small solid arrows). The ventricular system has been made radiolucent by introduction of gas (encephalography).

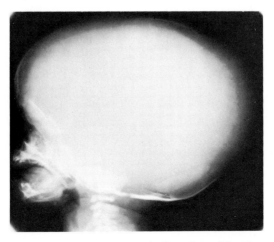

Fig. 4-27. The skull may increase in size. A markedly enlarged head is present at birth, in this case as a result of dilatation of the ventricles (hydrocephalus).

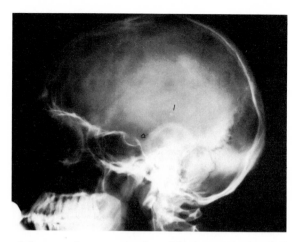

Fig. 4-28. Hydrocephalus may intervene in the adult; however, the skull can no longer increase in size because the sutures are closed. Effects of increased intracranial pressure are manifested by bony erosion. The dorsum sellae (open arrow) is affected. The pineal (solid arrow) lies in approximately the normal location, however.

The skull is a sphere and multiple projections are necessary for complete study. The views most frequently used are the lateral, P-A, A-P, and basal projections. Fig. 4-29 illustrates the various views.

PARANASAL SINUSES

The paranasal sinuses are divided into four groups: frontal, ethmoid, maxillary, and sphenoid. The standard projections used in filming the paranasal sinuses are shown in Figs. 4-30 to 4-33. The Caldwell projection shows the frontal and ethmoid sinuses to advantage. While the patient's forehead and nose rest on the film, the x-ray beam enters the back of his head perpendicular to the film. The lateral projection is used particularly for the frontal sinuses and the sphenoid sinuses. The alveolar recesses of the maxillary antra and ethmoid sinuses can be seen, although the right and left cells are superimposed one upon the other. When properly used the basal projection provides one of the best screening films for both the mastoids and the sinuses, but requires familiarity with the anatomic structures depicted. It is obtained with the head fully extended. The film is placed against the top of the head; the beam enters beneath the chin parallel to the long axis of the body. Superimposition of right and left sinus groups is avoided. The view most commonly referred to is the Waters projection. It is obtained with the nose and the chin of the patient resting against the film; the x-ray beam passes through the back of the head, perpendicular to the film. The Waters projection is similar to the Caldwell projection in that the anterior and posterior portions of the sinuses are superimposed; however, the right and left sinuses are seen separately in both of these projections.

The paranasal sinuses normally contain air and are radiolucent, in contrast to the surrounding bony envelopes. The sinuses are lined with mucosa. At the

Text continued on p. 222.

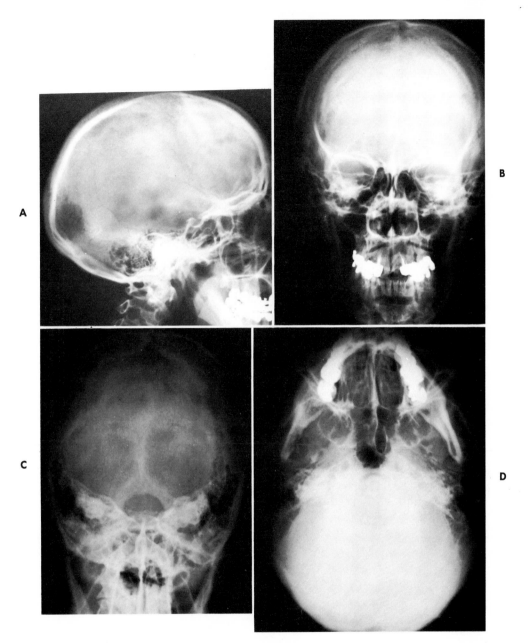

Fig. 4-29. A normal skull series usually consists of a minimum of four projections. **A,** The lateral view demonstrates the sella turcica and clinoid processes, calvarial structure, and mastoid aeration, and allows identification of anterior posterior migration of intracranial densities. **B,** The P-A projection gives a tangential look at parietal bone, facial structures, petrous ridges, and makes possible identification of right to left shift of intracranial densities. **C,** The Chamberlain-Towne view, done A-P with the head flexed 45°, allows a view of the posterior parietal bone tangentially, the occipital bone head on, the foramen magnum with posterior clinoids overlying, the petrous portion of temporal bone with density of labyrinthine structures and cochlea, and the ascending rami of mandible. **D,** The basal view shows the basilar foramina (ovale, spinosum, and magnum), petrous ridges, mastoid air cells, and paranasal sinuses.

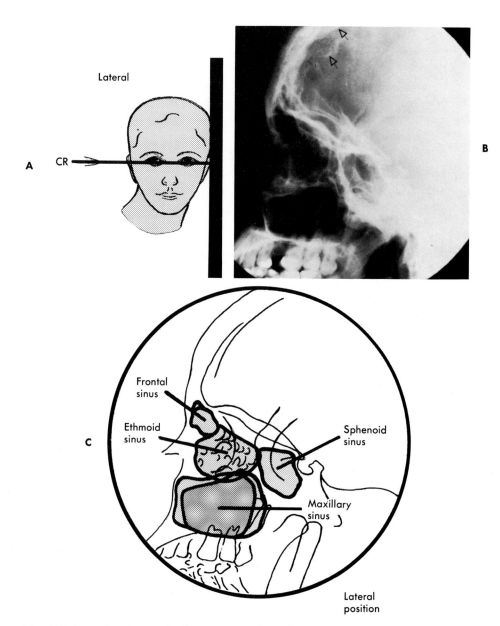

Fig. 4-30. Lateral projection. In this projection the right sinuses are superimposed on the left. The sphenoid sinuses and the posterior margins of the maxillary antra are well seen. A coincidental finding is moderate hyperostosis frontalis interna (open arrows). Notice that the sphenoid sinuses reach to the anterior wall of the sella turcica and that the roof of the air cells of the body of the sphenoid represents the planum sphenoidale. By following this line anteriorly the cribriform plate can be identified on the regular film. **A,** Head position showing passage of the central ray through the skull and relationship of head to film. **B,** Sinuses as seen on radiograph. **C,** Relative position of sinuses.

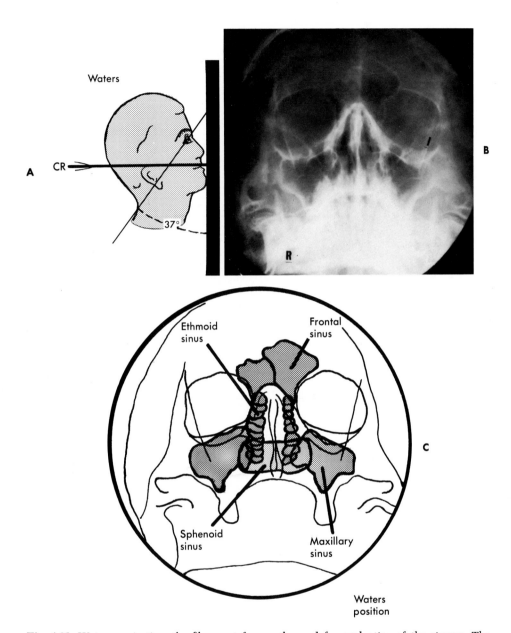

Fig. 4-31. Waters projection, the film most frequently used for evaluation of the sinuses. The outline of the sinuses is demonstrated by the shaded areas in **C.** The sphenoid, ethmoid, and maxillary sinuses overlap in the region of the inferior, medial aspect of the orbit. The oblique orbital line (*I*) is identifiable. This is the anterolateral margin of the orbit and is an important landmark in determining the status of the bony structure of the orbit. The superimposition of the anterior and posterior wall of the sinuses makes full evaluation of these areas somewhat difficult. **A,** Head position showing passage of central ray through the skull and the relationship of head to film. **B,** Sinuses as seen on radiograph. **C,** Relative position of sinuses.

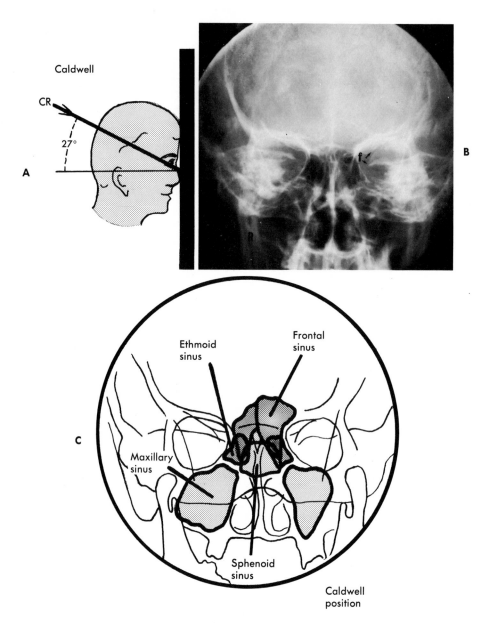

Fig. 4-32. Caldwell projection. The frontal sinuses are seen head on, and the sphenoidal sinuses are somewhat better seen in their lateral extent. The superior orbital fissure (*f*) is well identified. The petrous ridges are projected through the orbit and the mastoid air cells; the petrous tips, semicircular canals, and internal auditory canals are all identifiable. **A,** Head position showing passage of central ray through the skull and the relationship of head to film. **B,** Sinuses as seen on radiograph. **C,** Relative position of sinuses.

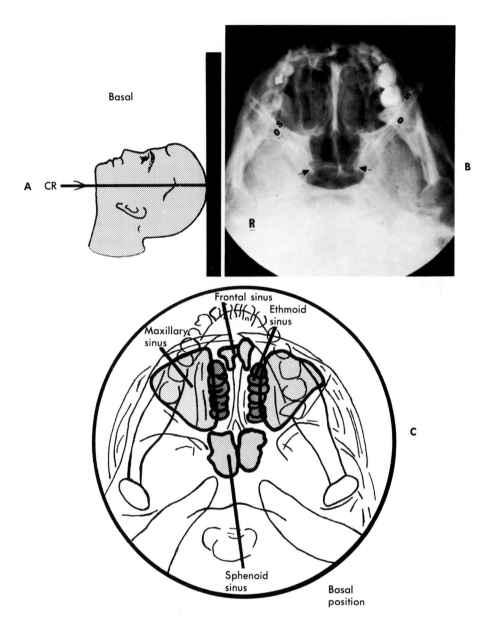

Fig. 4-33. The basal or submental vertical view. The maxillary antra are easily identified with their posterior wall (*s*) being shown as a sigmoid curved bony density. One of the bony margins of the orbit is also seen as a straight line (*o*). Lying between these two lines is the inferior orbital fissure. The frontal sinuses are seen as rather small air cells lying far anteriorly, with their anterior and posterior walls shown separately. The sphenoid sinuses are now seen without superimposition of other sinuses and with the right and left side being shown (solid arrows). Because this projection reduces much of the overlapping of the sinuses, it is one of the better survey films for the sinuses. **A,** Head position showing passage of central ray through the skull and the relationship of head to film. **B,** Sinuses as seen on radiograph. **C,** Relative position of sinuses.

junction of the mucous membrane and the bone is a very white line called the mucoperiosteal line. This landmark is used in tracing the extent of the sinuses. Poor definition of this line may result from abnormalities of the sinuses or the adjoining bone. As in the lung, since air is highly radiolucent, soft tissue irregu- larities in the sinuses are evident on the films. The most frequent roentgeno- graphic abnormality of the paranasal sinuses is soft tissue thickening of the mucosa (Figs. 4-34 and 4-35). The density of fluid from inflammation, submu- cosal retention cysts, and tumors is the same. The configuration of the density, however, does allow some differentiation. An air-fluid level is seen if the sinus is not completely opaque and if the patient is placed in the erect position at the time the film is made. The air-fluid level will shift with the head position. The soft tissue density of a solid tumor and the soft tissue density of a submucosal retention cyst can be distinguished by placing the patient's head in the lateral decubitus position. A difference in form may result with a change in the position of the head if a cyst is present. If, for an unknown reason, a sinus is totally opaque the status of the mucoperiosteal line becomes extremely important. If this line is well seen throughout, there is less likelihood that the soft tissue density repre- sents tumor. An opaque sinus in an older individual with loss of mucoperiosteal line and irregular radiolucency of adjoining bone should be considered evidence of tumor and definitive diagnostic measures taken (Fig. 4-36). The size, contour and location of the paranasal sinuses are highly variable. Communication with the air passageway during the formative years is needed for sinus development. Any obstructive lesions, such as mucosal edema at the site of the drainage ostea, may impair the aeration and growth of the paranasal sinuses. The paranasal

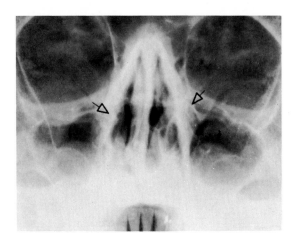

Fig. 4-34. Abnormality of the sinuses is usually demonstrated roentgenographically by reduced radiolucency as the result of loss of air. Rounded soft tissue densities (small solid arrows) lie in the floor of the maxillary antra bilaterally. These represent submucosal retention cysts from previous infection. The open arrows indicate that there is reduced aeration of the ethmoid sinuses as well.

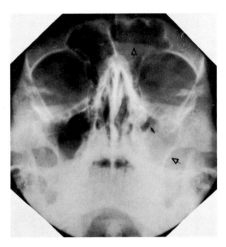

Fig. 4-35. Diffuse infection may be unilateral. An air-fluid level is present in the left frontal sinus (upper open arrow). The left maxillary antrum is totally opaque (lower open arrow). The apparent radiolucency (small solid arrow) is the overlying superior orbital fissure and does not represent aeration within the central portion of the sinus. The ethmoid sinuses also are abnormally dense.

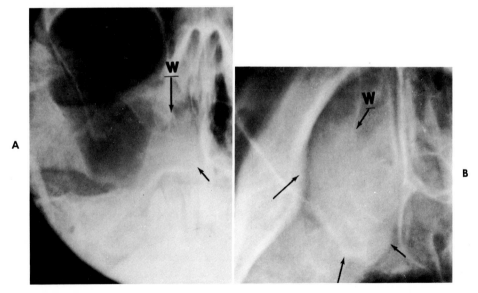

Fig. 4-36. The bony walls of the sinuses may be affected by disease. The medial wall of the maxillary antrum (W) is not identifiable because of destruction by cancer originating in the maxillary antrum. The posterior wall (long solid arrows, **B**) is also observed to be absent. A mass (short solid arrow, **A**, **B**) is seen projecting into the nasal passageway. **A**, The Waters projection shows that the inferior margin of the orbit is still present. **B**, The basal projection shows that the orbital line is not affected posteriorly but that the mass which projects into the nasal passageway approximates the midline. The ethmoid sinuses are poorly aerated as well, but the septa can be identified on the basal projection.

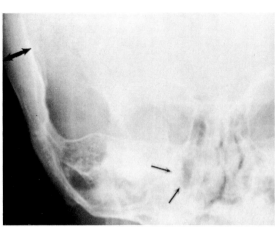
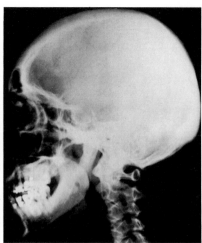

| Fig. 4-37 | Fig. 4-38 |

Fig. 4-37. Excess bone may produce increased density in the sinus areas. The calvarium is quite thick (broad double-ended arrow). The maxillary antrum is quite small (short solid arrows). The chronic anemia from which this patient suffers has caused a change in the structure of the bone of the maxilla preventing aeration.

Fig. 4-38. Change in paranasal sinus size may reflect hormonal influence. Hyperactivity of the anterior lobe of the pituitary causes acromegaly in the adult. In a classic example, the sella turcica is enlarged, with a thin anterior posterior diameter of the dorsum sellae. The frontal sinuses are large, the angle of the mandible is obtuse, and the calvarium is thick. The bone of the skull, while quite thick, is frequently rather poorly mineralized.

sinuses may be small if there is abnormality of the adjoining bone. One example is the individual suffering from anemia with excessive demand on the bone marrow of the maxilla (Fig. 4-37). This prevents invasion of the bone by the enlarging sinuses and produces a small sinus in adulthood. Some influence of hormones on the size of the sinuses exists but is as yet poorly understood. Acromegaly (hyperpituitarism, eosinophilic type) stimulates growth, particularly of the frontal sinuses (Fig. 4-38). Sinuses continue to increase in size throughout life, although at a rather slow rate compared to childhood.

The sinus cells grow both in their bone of origin and adjoining bones. Ethmoidal air cells, for example, are commonly present in the supraorbital portion of the frontal bone, the posterior aspect of the maxillae, and even the sphenoid. The usual roentgenographic study of the paranasal sinuses utilizes most of the parameters in order to clearly determine normality or abnormality. Thus, dense, small maxillary antra with relatively fine margination most likely result from inflammatory disease in childhood. Extensively developed, very well aerated paranasal sinuses may represent decreased cerebral growth, since this is one of the mechanisms utilized in occupying excess space in the natural development of the skull.

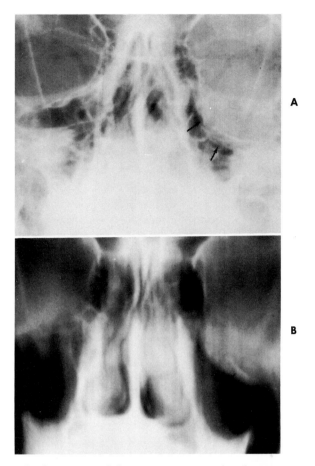

Fig. 4-39. Trauma to the face is one of the common reasons for obtaining views of the paranasal sinuses. A forceful blow to the orbit may cause a "blowout" fracture of the floor of the
orbit which is also the roof of the maxillary antrum. **A,** The Waters projection shows the
penetration of the orbital contents through a disrupted floor of the orbit on the left (arrows).
This produces a reduced aeration in the upper portion of the antrum as contrasted to the
normal right side. **B,** Tomography is valuable in demonstrating such fractures; the fractured
fragment of the floor of the orbit (solid arrow) is now well shown.

FACIAL BONES AND ORBITS

The delicate structure of these bones requires specialized roentgenographic
techniques in order to be adequately seen. Complete study of these bones often
requires tomography. Roentgenographic studies of the facial bones are usually
done to determine if a fracture is present following trauma. Fractures are
usually seen as radiolucent lines. If the margins of a fracture overlap, however, these will appear radiodense from the double thickness of cortex. If
the fracture involves the floor of the orbit, a "blow-out fracture" may result (Fig. 4-39). Increased density of the maxillary antrum is produced on
that side of the face. Sinusitis is the usual misdiagnosis in such a case. The

patient's history of trauma and epistaxis, however, should suggest a fracture and hemorrhage.

Increased density of the facial bones sometimes results from systemic osteo-sclerotic diseases. Healing inflammation or benign tumors, such as osteomas, may also cause hyperostosis (Fig. 4-40). The frontal sinuses and the mandible may be sites of osteomas.

The thinness of the facial bones makes it difficult to distinguish the reduced density of osteoporosis.

The orbits and the paranasal sinuses can be studied by artificially changing their density. The density of the orbit is usually artificially reduced by means of injection of air into the retro-orbital areas (pneumoorbitography). The muscle cone and soft tissues of the orbit are thereby shown. By selectively opacifying the vessels leading to the orbits the density is artificially increased. Opacification of the paranasal sinuses is achieved by direct instillation of iodinated compounds (Fig. 4-41). This technique is useful for differentiating causes of intrasinus densities. Abnormal densities may occur in the orbits (Fig. 4-42).

The size of the orbits is dependent upon the character of the surrounding bones. If there is good growth potential and the contained structures or spaces are normal in volume, the growth of the orbits and sinuses will be normal. Increased amount of intraorbital tissues, such as hemangiomas, may produce an abnormally large orbit. Conversely, if the eye is damaged and fails to grow or is removed at an early age, the orbit will be small. The orbit is normally quite large.

The orbits normally have a predictable location; however, variations in development occur. An increased or a decreased distance between the orbits results.

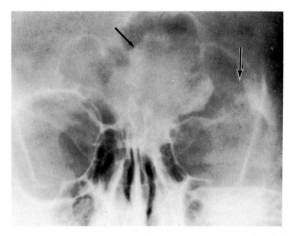

Fig. 4-40. Benign tumors may originate in the sinuses. An irregular lobulated density, an osteoma (small arrow), lies within the frontal sinuses. This is reactive bone formation caused by previous infection. The left supraorbital ridge is absent (outlined arrow) as the result of surgery for infection of the frontal sinuses.

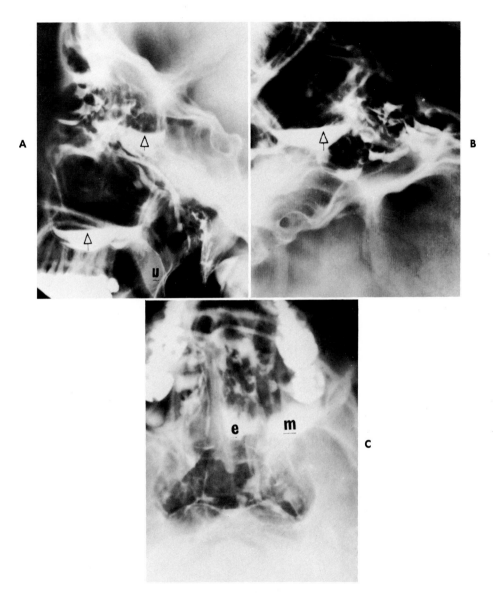

Fig. 4-41. An artificial change in density of the paranasal sinuses is accomplished by introducing an iodinated compound. This demonstrates the status of the lining of the sinuses. The location of the sinuses is also identified. **A,** In the erect lateral projection air-fluid levels are apparent; the upper arrow shows the posterior cellular structure of the ethmoids and the lower arrow the floor of the maxillary antra. The uvula (*u*) is coated with contrast medium posteriorly and is contrasted against the air of the oropharynx anteriorly. **B,** With the patient lying on her back the contrast medium gravitates to the more dependent portions of the sinuses. The open arrow shows the posterior superior margin of the maxillary antrum; its area of overlap of the posterior ethmoidal cells is well seen. The multiple cellular structure of the ethmoids is well depicted. **C,** With the patient lying on her back and the beam projected in a submental vertex projection, the posterior margins of the ethmoids (*e*) are seen as well as the posterior recess of the maxillary antrum (*m*). This is a normal study.

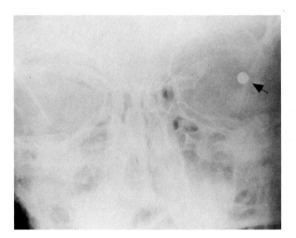

Fig. 4-42. Accidental introduction of increased density in this instance results from an air rifle pellet that has penetrated the left eye (solid arrow). Roentgenography enables very accurate localization of foreign bodies within the eye to assist in their surgical removal.

Fig. 4-43. Specific views of the optic foramina are used to determine normality. **A,** The films are made with the head positioned as diagrammed. These utilize the contrasting air, bone, and soft tissues. The usual appearance is seen in **B.** Identification of the various anatomic structures, **C,** shows that the zygoma (*z*) forms the lateral margin of the orbit. The superior orbital fissure (*f*) is set off from the optic foramen (*o*) by the sphenoidal strut (solid arrow). The anterior clinoid (*c*) projects posteriorly from the optic foramen. The planum sphenoidale (*p*) angles to the viewer's right, reaching anteriorly to the level of the cribriform plate. The ethmoidal air cells (*e*) overlie the medial anterior aspect of the orbit, with the maxillary antrum (*m*) shown as overlapping the posterior ethmoidal area. **D,** Abnormality of the optic foramen is manifested by an increase in its diameter. In this case it is a physiologic variation, since the bony strut is intact; however, it is quite large, measuring 6.1 by 5.6 mm. **E,** The Waters projection provides an evaluation of the orbital structures. The oblique orbital line (*I*) delineates the anterolateral wall of the orbit. The zygomatic prominence and frontal process of the zygoma (*z*) are the most anterolateral aspects of the bony orbit. The posterior superior medial aspect of the orbit is assessable by the relative definition of the superior orbital fissure (*f*) and the superior aspect of the posterior ethmoidal group (*e*). The anterior clinoid (*c*) now overlies the medial aspect of the orbit and the planum sphenoidale (*p*) is riding upward and anteriorly toward the viewer. The maxillary antrum (*m*) provides the floor of the orbit. The sphenoid sinuses occasionally become quite large (*s*), extending well out into the sphenoidal wing; they may pneumatize the lesser wing of the sphenoid. The structures labeled on the right are identifiable on the left and can be used to study the normal roentgenographic appearance.

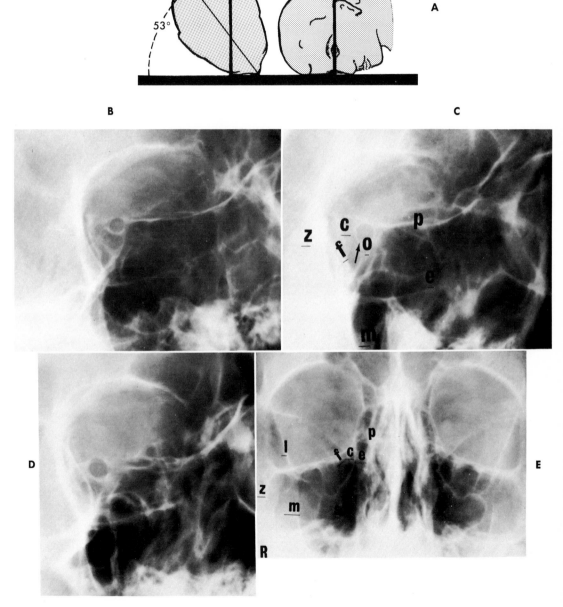

Fig. 4-43. For legend see opposite page.

The location of the nasal septum and the nasal bones makes them susceptible to trauma and developmental variation.

The following bony landmarks assist in identifying the margins of the orbit:

1. Linea innominata (oblique orbital line), lateral wall of orbit
2. Superior and inferior orbital fissures seen on the Caldwell and basal projections, frequently confused with posterior ethmoid air cells and sphenoid sinus
3. Optic foramina lying quite far posteriorly and entering the orbit at an oblique angle.
4. Fossa for the lacrimal gland lying in the superior lateral portion of the orbit and identifiable as a crescentic hyperostotic area.
5. Infraorbital foramen

The infraorbital foramen migrates during life and eventually, if sinus development is normal, presents in the infraorbital ridge. If the sinuses do not develop well, this foramen will remain in its infantile position in the upper part of the maxilla. The foramen rotundum is best seen on the Caldwell or the Waters projection. The intactness of the anterior floor of the middle fossa can be determined in part by the appearance of the foramen rotundum. The sphenoid bone plays an important role in the structures of the skull. The superior orbital fissures are surrounded by portions of the sphenoid bone. The vidian canal traverses the sphenoid bone. Foramina rotundi, spinosi, ovale, and optic foramina, are all within the sphenoids. The internal carotid arteries enter the skull lateral to the body of the sphenoid. They course medially to the anterior clinoids in close apposition to the sella turcica (Fig. 4-43).

TEMPORAL BONE

The temporal bone deserves specific consideration because of its complexity. Roentgenographic study of the abnormalities of the temporal bone is usually of the mastoids, the middle ear, and the internal auditory meatus. The extreme denseness of the cortical bone surrounding the labyrinthine structures, the obliquity of the petrous ridges, the skull, and the complexity of the structures make roentgenographic examination of this area difficult.

MASTOIDS

Certain projections are commonly used in the examination of the mastoids. These include the Law's projection (the head is placed in the lateral position), the Chamberlain-Towne projection (the head is flexed approximately 45° and the beam is directed through the forehead and exits through the region of the foramen magnum), the basal projection (similar to the view for demonstration of the paranasal sinuses, providing one of the best survey films of the mastoids), and the Stenvers projection (the patient is in a prone position with the head turned 45° toward the side to be studied).

Understanding the anatomy of the mastoids requires knowledge of positioning. In the series illustrated in Figs. 4-44 through 4-49, diagrammatic representation of the position of the head and the course of the central x-ray beam

Text continued on p. 236.

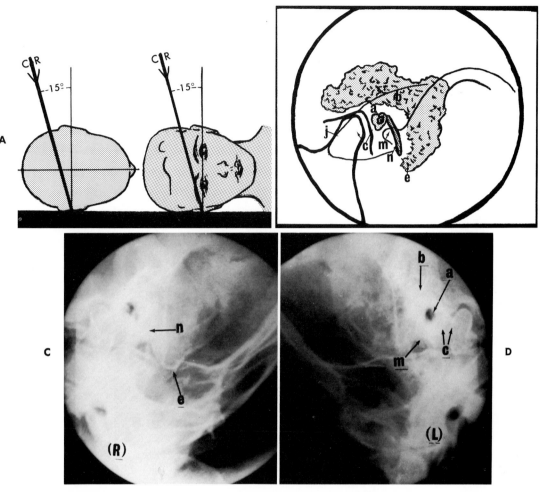

Fig. 4-44. Law's projections. The normal ossicles (*a*) lie below the antrum (*b*) and in the tympanic cavity which lies above the jugular fossa (*m*). Aerated mastoid cells are present in **D** in contrast to the sclerotic cells from infection in **C**. The facial canal (*n*) in **C**, however, is somewhat better seen. The mastoid tip (*e*) in **C** stands out because of the sclerosis.

In the following illustrations:

A is a diagram of the head-film position used in making the radiographs. **B** is a diagrammatic representation of the anatomy seen on the films. The lighter stippled areas represent aerated structures. Darker stippling outlines either vascular or neural structures. CR represents the central x-ray beam. The following key applies to Figs. 4-44 through 4-49.

Key to labeled anatomy

a Ossicles
b Mastoid antrum
c Eustachian tube and condyle of the mandible
d Carotid artery canal
e Mastoid tip
f Root of zygoma
g Sphenoid sinus
h Margins of internal auditory canal

i Stylomastoid foramen (basal projection)
j Superior margin of the petrous ridge (see Low-Beer projection)
k Arcuate eminence (over semicircular canals)
l Crista falciformis (see Low-Beer projections)
m Jugular fossa (see Law's projection)
n Facial canal (see Law's projection)
o Cochlea

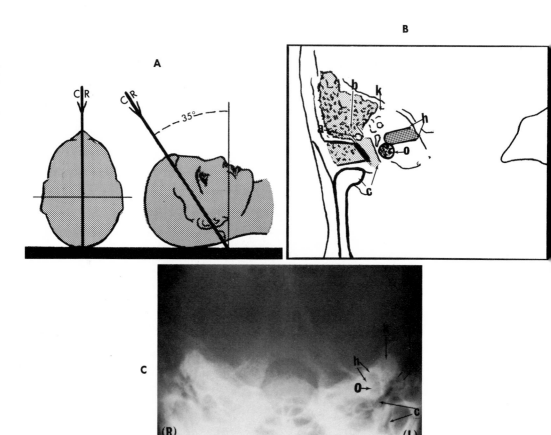

Fig. 4-45. Chamberlain-Towne projection. **C,** The eustachian tube (*c*) lying medial to the condyle of the mandible leads to the region of the tympanic cavity, where the ossicles rest. The parallel lines extending up and laterally indicate the margins of the aditus, the passage of the air into the mastoid antrum (*b*). The semicircular canals are seen underneath the arcuate eminence (*k*) lying posterior and lateral to the internal auditory canal (*h*). Lying inferior to the internal auditory canal is the cochlea (*o*). The aditus and ossicles on the right are poorly seen as the result of the disease process. (See Fig. 4-44 for key.)

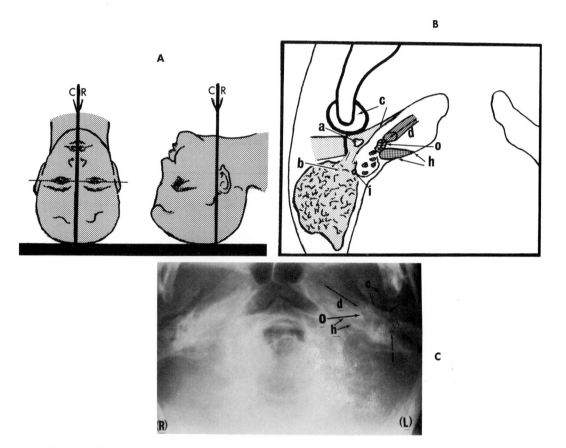

Fig. 4-46. Basal projection. **C,** The eustachian tube and condyle of the mandible (*c*) are well seen leading to the tympanic cavity containing the ossicles (*a*). Extending posteriorly and laterally from the area of the tympanic cavity (parallel lines) is the aditus, leading to the mastoid antrum (*b*). The stylomastoid foramen (*i*) lies just slightly posterior and medial to the aditus. The carotid canal (*d*) is now seen extending through the petrous tip. Just posterior to this is the internal auditory canal (*h*). The cochlea (*o*) lies between the carotid canal and the internal auditory canal. The left side is normal, whereas the right side shows loss of ossicles and loss of definition of the aditus, indicative of cholesteatoma formation. (See Fig. 4-44 for key.)

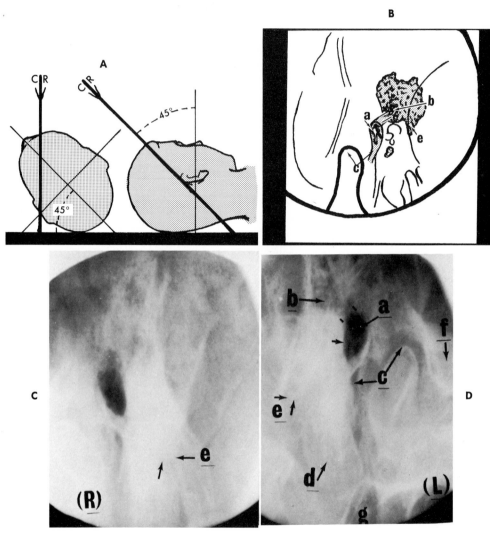

Fig. 4-47. C, D, The Owens (modified Mayer) projection shows the ossicles (*a*) lying within the tympanic cavity. Air has reached the tympanic cavity by way of the eustachian tube (middle arrow, *c*), which lies parallel to the temporomandibular fossa and the condyle of the mandible (upward pointing arrow, *c*). From here the air passes through the aditus (parallel lines) to enter the mastoid antrum (*b*). Lying between the parallel lines is a fine white line that represents the bony bridge. The mastoid tip is rotated medially (*e*), with the carotid canal coming from the petrous tip (*d*). The sphenoid sinus is identified as lying inferiorly (*g*) and the root of the zygoma laterally (*f*). In **C** there is absence of the bony bridge, and the major portion of the ossicles and loss of definition of the mastoid antrum and aditus as the result of cholesteatoma. (See Fig. 4-44 for key.)

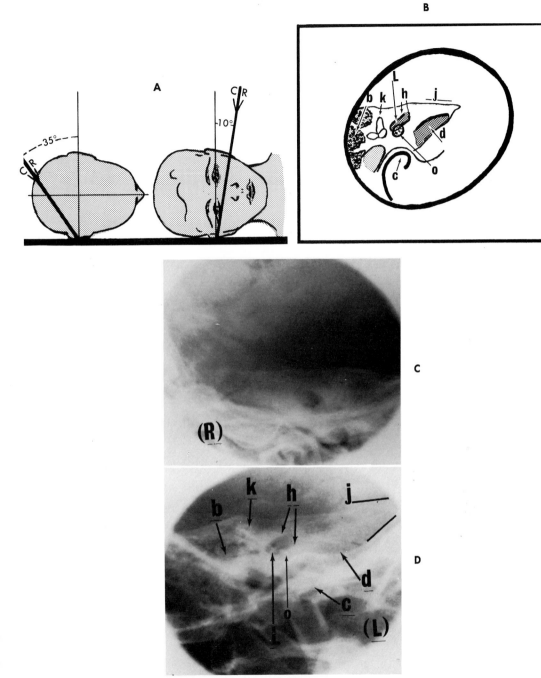

Fig. 4-48. Low-Beer projection. **C** represents the diseased right side with loss of definition in the region of the mastoid antrum. **D,** shows the normal side with the mastoid antrum (*b*) lying posterolaterally to the semicircular canals which lie under the arcuate eminence (*k*). The internal auditory canal (*h*), containing the cochlea (*o*) with the crista falciformis as its roof (*L*), is well shown in this projection. Immediately above this is a small round hole that represents passage of the facial nerve through the internal auditory canal. The tip of the petrous ridge angles to the right (*j*); its lower margin is defined by the black line. The condyle of the mandible is seen (*c*) lying inferior to the area of the carotid canal (*d*). (See Fig. 4-44 for key.)

is depicted. The resulting roentgenograms are illustrated, and diagrammatic representation of the major structures is shown. In the roentgenograms the left side is normal and the right side demonstrates the result of chronic infection and cholesteatoma formation. A cholesteatoma is a small tumor-like growth which may develop within a chronically infected ear if the eardrum is perforated.

Three lines of reference are usable in studying mastoids:

1. The line of aeration includes the eustachian tube, tympanic cavity, aditus, and mastoid antrum. (Owens projection *c-a-b* [Fig. 4-47], Chamberlain-Towne projection *c-b* [Fig. 4-45], basal projection *c-a-b* [Fig. 4-46].)

2. The line of sound includes the external canal, tympanic membrane, tympanic cavity and ossicles, and internal auditory meatus. (Chamberlain-

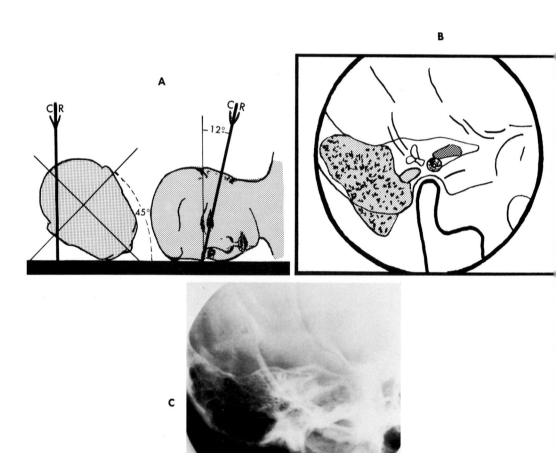

Fig. 4-49. Stenvers projection. **C,** This is a normal film, showing essentially the same anatomy demonstrated on the Low-Beer projection except that the petrous ridge is shortened and the internal auditory canals are somewhat rounder.

Towne projection [Fig. 4-45], external canal through *h;* basal projection [Fig. 4-46], external canal *a-h.*)

3. The paracentral line is visible on the basal projection only [Fig. 4-45] and represents the line parallel to the sagittal plane of the skull with its anterior anchor in the foramen spinosum. It includes the foramen spinosum (just medial to *c*), the eustachian tube (*c*), the lateral aspect carotid canal (*d*), the cochlea (*o*), the lateral portion internal auditory canal (*h*), and the jugular fossa.

Inflammation in the mastoids produces similar changes to those seen in the paranasal sinuses. The lack of aeration at an early age prevents development of normal air cell size. Well-developed mastoids usually contain a moderate quantity of air. Edema (mucosal swelling) or exudate (fluid from inflammation) produces loss of aeration and increased roentgenographic density of the mastoids. The walls that set off the small mastoid air cells (septa) may be lost in infection. The thinned septae may still be seen at an early phase of the disease. If infection persists, the septae will resorb and an overall haziness of the mastoids results (Fig. 4-50). An increased density (hyperostotic response) is visible if mastoid infection occurred at an early age (Fig. 4-51). The cells may fail to develop satisfactorily if some obstruction occurred in childhood and diploic-type bone is present in the mastoids.

Air reaches the mastoids by way of the eustachian tubes. Obstruction of this tube at the time of mastoid development may preclude pneumatization of the mastoids. Stenosis of the eustachian tube occasionally produces decreased aeration and size of the tympanic cavity and mastoids; as a result the density of the mastoids is increased.

Infection is the usual cause for bony destruction which causes abnormally re-

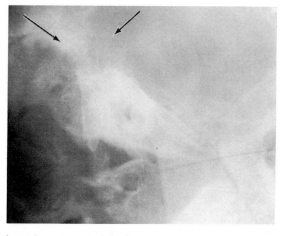

Fig. 4-50. There is loss of aeration and bony septation of the mastoid air cells in the region of the mastoid antrum (arrows). It is loss of bony density and reduced radiolucency of aeration that indicate abnormal tissue, in this instance, acute infection.

duced density. Cholesteatomas may form in chronically infected ears. Erosion of
the bone by pressure of the growing mass may be seen roentgenographically in
the middle ear. A similar effect is produced by granulation tissue in the middle
ear. The density of the tympanic cavity can be artificially altered by contrast
medium passed into the middle ear by way of the eustachian tubes.

The size of the mastoids, petrous ridges, internal auditory meatus and otic
structures is quite variable from individual to individual and from side to side.
Thickening of the calvarium, increase in size of the paranasal sinuses, and increased size of mastoid air cells may reflect poorly developed brain substance.

Margination. Extension of infection or abnormality into the adjoining osseous
structure may cause loss of distinct margination of the mastoid air cells. Occasionally, aberrant cells may appear as unusual lucencies. The periantral, lateral,
tip, zygomatic, posterior, paratubal, and squamosal cells constitute the various
air cells of the mastoid.

The otic capsule is the most dense cortical bone in the body. Lying within
this dense capsule are the semicircular canals, vestibule, and cochlea (the labyrinth). Once identified, these provide excellent landmarks for interpretation of
roentgenograms. The cochlea's close apposition to the internal auditory canal
assists in locating the canal on roentgenograms. The internal auditory canal is
normally sharply defined. Normal pneumatization of the petrous tip or osteoporosis may blur the margins of the canal. Bone destruction by inflammatory disease
or tumor of the eighth cranial nerve may cause loss of form and increased size
of the internal auditory meatus (Fig. 4-52). The mastoids are prone to hyperostotic response from previous infection. Sufficient new bone may form to involve
the middle ear and decrease the aeration of the tympanic cavity. Inflammation
of the petrous tip may also cause hyperostosis and produce narrowing of the

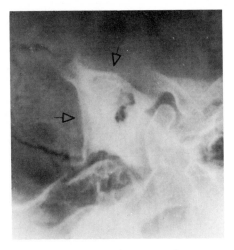

Fig. 4-51. Inflammatory disease of the mastoids can produce excessive bone density as the
result of hyperostotic response as part of the healing phase. This is evident along the course
of the sinus plate (lower open arrow) and tegmen (upper open arrow).

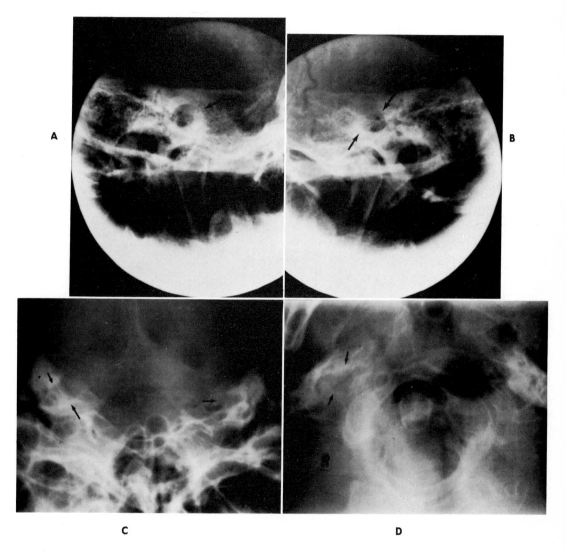

Fig. 4-52. Loss of bony substance and increased size indicates erosion. **A,** The Low-Beer projection shows a tumor (arrow) of the internal auditory meatus, which is seen to be enlarged when compared to the normal size (**B,** apposing arrows). **C,** The Chamberlain-Towne projection shows enlargement of the canal on the right (opposing arrows) as compared to the normal canal on the left (single arrow). **D,** On the basal projection the widening of the medial aspect of the internal auditory canal (apposing arrows) is contrasted with the normal canal on the left (single arrow).

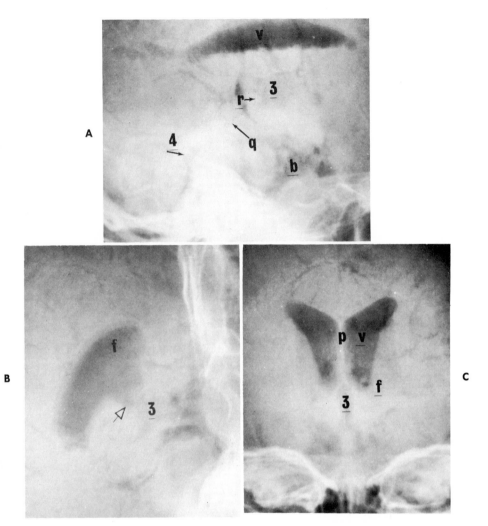

Fig. 4-53. Gas introduced into the lumbar subarachnoid space is allowed to rise through the spinal canal to define the ventricular structures of the brain. **A,** In the erect position the gas first reaches the fourth ventricle (*4*), then passes through the aqueduct of Sylvius (*q*) to reach the third ventricle (*3*). As viewed in the lateral projection the pineal recess (*r*) projects into the posterior part of the third ventricle, with the body of the lateral ventricle lying above the third ventricle (*v*). The basal cisterns (*b*) are also defined, in this instance, at the level of the stalk of the hypophysis. **B,** With the patient lying on his back and viewed on the lateral projection, the gas collects in the frontal horns of the lateral ventricles (*f*) and outlines the foramen of Monro (open arrow), which communicates with the third ventricle (*3*). **C,** The film taken at right angles with the beam passing from the forehead through the occiput shows the midline position of the third ventricle (*3*), the body of the lateral ventricles (*v*), and the frontal horn (*f*). Separating the right and left lateral ventricles is the septum pellucidum (*p*). **D,** With the patient in the prone position gas rises to the occipital horns (*o*) and defines the posterior bodies of the lateral ventricles. **E,** In the P-A projection the posterior ventricular system, including the fourth ventricle (*4*) and the occipital horns of the lateral ventricle (*o*), are noted. Some gas has collected in the cerebellopontine angle cistern (*cp*). This is considered a normal study.

internal auditory canal. Compression of the nerve and reduced hearing may result.

The contour of the structures of the ear is predictable. The middle ear cavity is lens-shaped. The internal auditory meatus has a juglike contour in its vertical dimension. The petrous tips have a rounded inferior margin. Alterations in these various forms may be normal variations or the primary clues to an abnormality.

The three ossicles—the malleus, incus, and stapes—are in the middle ear. Displacement of the ossicles occurs in trauma, infection, or tumor. They may be destroyed by infection or tumor; or they may fail to become differentiated during embryonic development. The aditus leads from the middle ear to the mastoid antrum. The margination of the aditus is an important clue in detecting inflammatory disease of the middle ear. Tumors of the nasopharynx may cause erosion of the inferior aspect of the petrous tip reducing the sharpness of its margins.

INTRACRANIAL STRUCTURES

The largest intracranial structures are nerve tissues (the brain, cranial nerves, and medulla oblongata). Other structures provide nourishment and support for the nervous system. The normal intracranial structures are of soft tissue density and not identifiable on the routine roentgenograms.

The density may be altered naturally by calcification. Calcification is most common in the pineal. The pineal gland thus provides an important landmark in determining normality of size and configuration of the intracranial structures, since its usual position is well charted. Calcifications are frequently seen in the dura, arteries, and choroidal plexus and occasionally occur in tumors of neural

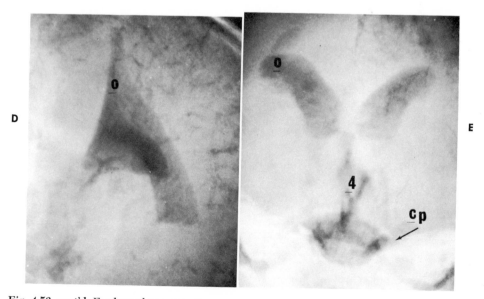

Fig. 4-53, cont'd. For legend see opposite page.

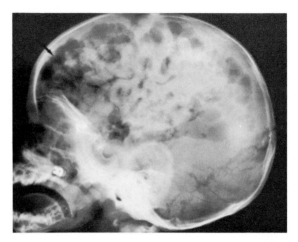

Fig. 4-54. In contrast to the normal subarachnoid space there is gross enlargement of the normal channels and irregular collections of gas beneath the arachnoid resulting from cerebral atrophy (arrow).

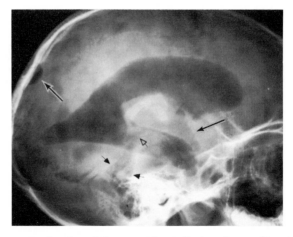

Fig. 4-55. An increase in the size of the ventricles indicates abnormality. Air has been introduced directly through a needle inserted into the ventricles by means of a bur hole (posterior solid arrow) placed in the skull. This demonstrates the enlarged lateral ventricle and enlarged third ventricle (anterior solid arrow) with the gas passing through the aqueduct of Sylvius (open arrows) to define an enlarged fourth ventricle (apposing solid arrows). Obstruction to the flow of cerebrospinal fluid, resulting from a cyst in the posterior fossa, has produced dilatation.

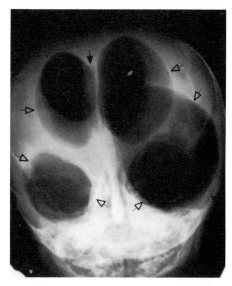

Fig. 4-56. Dilatation of the ventricles may be huge, as is demonstrated by the outline of the lateral ventricles (open arrows). An accessory ventricle (cavum septum pellucidum, solid arrow) lies between the lateral ventricles. The enlarged temporal horns overlie the orbits of the skull.

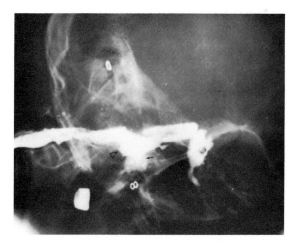

Fig. 4-57. Instead of gas, a radiopaque iodinated compound may be introduced into the posterior fossa to demonstrate the internal auditory canal (small solid arrow). The external canal on the side being examined is represented by the figure 8. The cerebellopontine angle cistern is also opacified (open arrow). Films are obtained with the patient lying on his side with the part to be examined dependent and with the petrous ridge perpendicular to the plane of viewing.

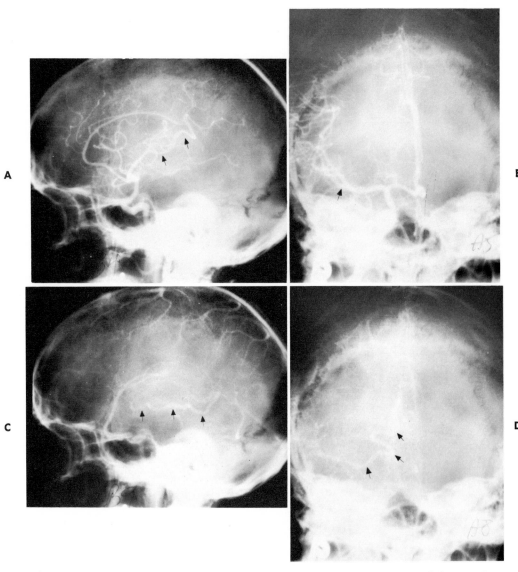

Fig. 4-58. Change in contrast, increased with either iodinated compound or radiolucency by air, affords information in tumor studies. **A,** Injection of contrast medium into the arteries on the lateral projection shows elevation of the middle cerebral artery (arrows). **B,** The Sylvian group which is seen in the A-P projection shows that the middle cerebral artery (arrow) is elevated laterally over the region of the temporal lobe. After the contrast medium has passed through the brain it re-collects in the venous structures, showing elevation of the basilar vein of Rosenthal on the lateral projection (**C,** arrows) and in the A-P projection (**D,** arrows). **E,** Pneumoencephalography demonstrates in the supine position amputation of the temporal horn (solid arrow) as seen in the lateral projection. **F,** In the A-P projection the temporal horn on the right (small arrow) is shown to be elevated and overlying a tumor mass as contrasted to the normal left side. The third ventricle is deviated to the left (double arrows), showing that the tumor lies on the right.

origin and vascular tumors. The pattern of calcification may reflect the cell type of the structure or tumor.

Artificially induced contrast is usually required to demonstrate the form of the structures of the brain. Reduced contrast is produced by injection of air into the lumbar subarachnoid space. The air rises through the spinal canal, passes through the foramina of Luschka and Magendie, enters the ventricular system, and defines the ventricles (pneumoencephalography) (Figs. 4-53 to 4-56). Air can also be introduced by drilling holes in the skull and placing a needle directly into the ventricles (ventriculography). The size, location, and form of the ventricles permit detection of excess tissue (tumors), loss of tissues (atrophy), loss of the usual channels over the brain (meningitis), or increased superficial convolutions (atrophy) (See Figs. 4-53 to 4-56). The air can be manipulated into the various portions of the ventricular system by turning the head.

Artificial positive density using the same substance as is used for myelography demonstrates the fourth ventricle, the aqueduct of Sylvius, and the posterior basilar cisterns (Fig. 4-57).

With positive or negative contrast, the parameters utilized remain the same. Increased volume of the ventricular structures results from reduced surrounding brain tissue, which is mainly caused by hydrocephaly and atrophy. Congenital malformation with absence of portions of the brain tissue alters the size and configuration of ventricular structures. Contrast studies correlated with plain film study of the skull allow comparison of brain size and overall size of the skull.

The compressibility of the brain makes possible ventricular system deformity from an abnormality at some distance. A frontal lobe tumor, for instance, may

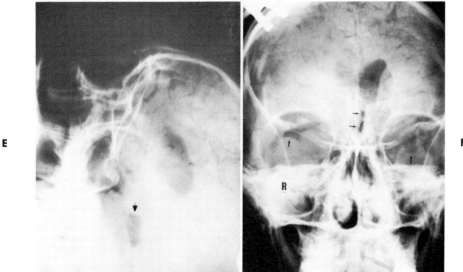

Fig. 4-58, cont'd. For legend see opposite page.

deform both the anterior frontal horn on the side of the lesion and the body of the lateral ventricle on the same side (Fig. 4-58).

Location of the intracranial structures is another major parameter. Loss of tissue on one side causes displacement of the ventricular and the midline structures toward the side of atrophy by the normal tissue on the other side. Some dilatation and distortion of the ventricles usually accompany atrophy. Displacement by excess tissue, as from tumor, usually produces some decrease in ventricular size and concomitant ventricular deformity. The pineal gland usually lies in the midline. Displacement of the pineal is one of the early clues to intracranial abnormality. On contrast studies, the septum pellucidum may also be altered in location and contour as the result of intracranial disease.

The number of subarachnoid basal cisterns may be altered by factitial lack of filling; however, unilateral absence of filling should suggest a pathologic condition. Accessory ventricles will occasionally develop in the septum pellucidum and fill with air during ventriculography or encephalography.

VASCULAR STRUCTURES

The brain is extremely sensitive to ischemia (lack of oxygen). Extensive vascular channels are present throughout the cranial vault. In roentgenographic studies, the course, location, size, number, and configuration of the arterial and venous channels are used in determining normality. The vessels are normally of soft tissue density and not identifiable on the routine films. Normal increased density (calcification) occurs frequently in the arterial wall (Fig. 4-59). Calcification from atherosclerosis may also be present in aneurysms or vascular fistulas.

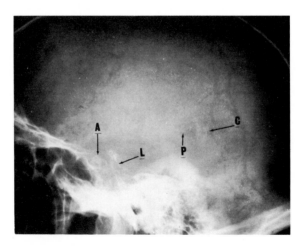

Fig. 4-59. Multiple areas of calcification normally occur within the skull as a result of aging. The area of choroidal pelxus calcification (*C*) is fairly large. The right and left side superimpose in this lateral projection. The pineal is faintly calcified (*P*) just anterior to the choroidal plexus lying in its normal location. The petroclinoid ligament (*L*) extends from the posterior clinoids to the petrous ridge. Calcification is present in the internal carotid arteries (*A*) and lies over the margin of the sella.

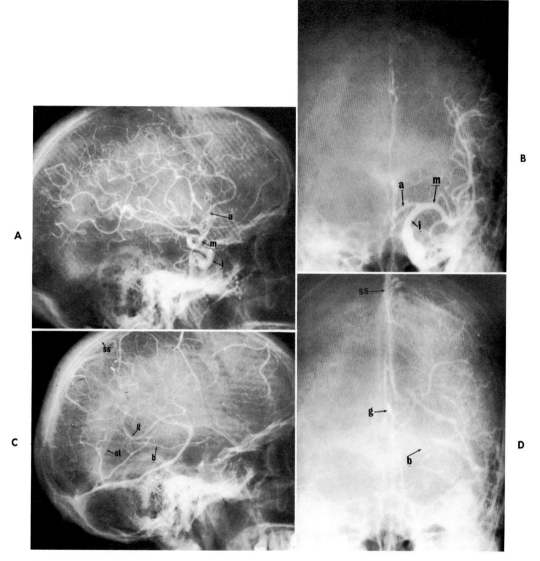

Fig. 4-60. In contrast to a distorted anatomy in an earlier study, the normal anatomy is shown in both the arterial and venous phases after injection of contrast medium into the arterial tree. It enters the skull through the internal carotid artery (*i*) as it passes through the foramen lacerum and divides into the anterior and middle cerebral arteries (*a* and *m*). These structures are identifiable on the lateral (**A**) and the A-P projection (**B**). **C,** The contrast medium defines the fine vessels of the brain and returns through the venous structures, subsequently outlining the sagittal sinus (*ss*), the great vein of Galen (*g*), the straight sinus (*st*), and the basilar vein of Rosenthal (*b*). **D,** The vein of Galen and sagittal sinus are midline, nonpaired structures, as is the straight sinus, while other structures are paired.

Artificially induced positive contrast is the most frequent method of satisfactory study of the vascular structures. An iodinated compound is injected either through a needle placed directly into the artery or vein, or through a catheter placed in the aortic arch by way of the arteries of the arm or thigh. Multiple rapid sequence films are used in at least two projections to determine the degree of filling, location, and size of the various vascular structures. The early films demonstrate the arterial tree and the delayed films the venous channels (Fig. 4-60).

Size. The size of the arterial and venous channels is highly variable. Spasm or thickening of the lining of the arteries decreases the size in contrast to the normal tapering of the arteries seen in the distal branches (Fig. 4-61). Focal dilatation of an artery may occur (aneurysm formation). A prominent arterial channel may lead to a tumor or unusual arteriovenous shunt. If a cause for excess arterial vascularity exists in one region, the veins leading from this region may have increased diameter.

Number. The intracranial vessels are usually paired structures, except for the basilar artery and the large midline venous sinuses. Incomplete demonstration of a vessel on one side may reflect intrinsic abnormality of that vessel or the surrounding tissues, or temporary spasm. Repeated injections will differentiate between spasm and other causes. Tumor formation or malformation of blood vessels may cause an excess number of vessels in one area (Fig. 4-62). The form of these differs from normal vessels. Congenital variations in numbers also occur (Fig. 4-63). The apparent number of vessels may be reduced either by obstruction of the vessel, as by thickening of the walls, or by spasm.

Contour. Deformity of the soft tissues from abnormalities of the brain will produce distortion of the course of the arteries or the veins. The vascular struc-

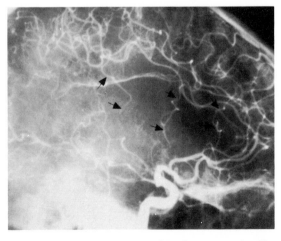

Fig. 4-61. Occlusion of the arterial tree may stimulate formation of collateral circulation (arrows). There is lack of filling of the middle cerebral artery as the result of clot formation.

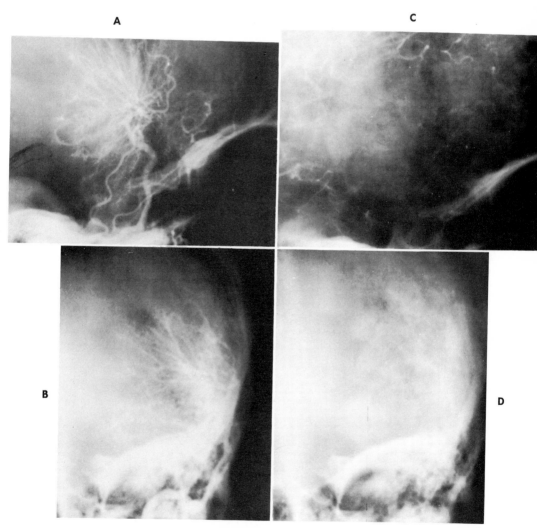

Fig. 4-62. Artificial opacification of specific vessels can demonstrate certain diseases. The injection of contrast medium into the external carotid, in this instance, opacifies a large, highly vascular tumor. **A,** In the lateral projection it is observed to lie immediately above the sella turcica. **B,** In the A-P projection the arterial phase shows that it extends posteriorly, superiorly, and inferiorly and lies far in the periphery. Subsequently, after venous filling has occurred as seen on the lateral projection (**C**) a diffuse density occurs which is better appreciated in the A-P projection (**D**) of the venous phase. This represents tumor blush and is very common in meningioma.

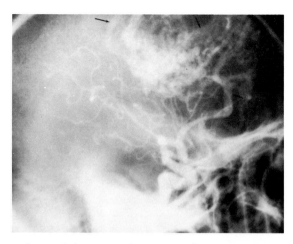

Fig. 4-63. Excess vessels may be present. The arrows indicate communication between arterial and venous phase opacification as the result of internal carotid arterial injection. This represents an arteriovenous malformation in the frontal portion of the brain. The veins opacify too rapidly as the result of the excess shunt.

tures tend to be displaced away from such abnormalities. The opacified arteries are primarily surface arteries, and their contour reflects the contour of the brain. Excess soft tissue beneath the skull, as in subdural hematoma, produces arterial distortion. The three-dimensional concept of the intracranial structures is important since a contour deformation may result from pressure from any direction. In the study of the cerebral vascularity, the vascular channels as a whole should be examined. No attempt is made to give a detailed anatomic review of the multiple arteries and veins. The reader is referred to well-established texts for this information.

The location of the arteries and veins in relation to the skull and to each other is predictable. Some displacement of the vessels can occur without appreciable distortion of contour. The position relative to the midline of the centrally located paired arterial structures and central venous sinuses is an important parameter. Displacement or retraction to one side is discernible when the films are obtained with the beam directed through the skull and parallel to the sagittal plane of the skull. Displacement from an expected location may be caused by excess or reduced amount of tissue on one side. Deformity of contour and displacement of the blood vessels is a sensitive indicator of abnormal form of the brain.

The margination of the blood vessels should be sharp. If modern techniques are used, there is usually rather complete filling of the blood vesesls by the bolus of contrast material. The streaming effect observed in the large peripheral arteries, aorta, and venous channels is not a major factor. Loss of sharp margination of the contrast bolus suggests rupture of the blood vessel and hemorrhage or extravasation of the contrast medium beyond the confines of the blood vessel. Irregularity of the wall comes from atheromatous calcific plaque or clot forma-

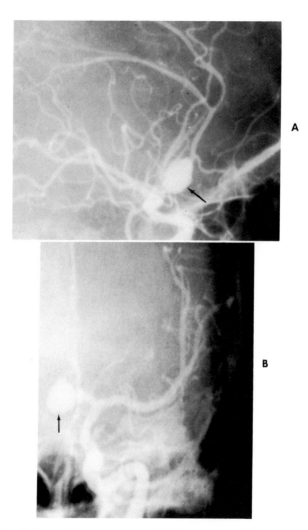

Fig. 4-64. The size of the vessels may increase. In this instance, there is a saccular dilatation (aneurysm, solid arrow) of the communicating artery between the anterior cerebral arteries as seen on the lateral (**A**) and in the A-P projection (**B**). The aneurysm is noted to lie slightly to the opposite side of the midline from the side of injection.

tion. A large portion of the sac of an aneurysm may be occupied by clot and not be opacified since the entrance of the contrast medium into the sac is prevented (Fig. 4-64).

REQUIRED READINGS

Caffey, J.: Pediatric x-ray diagnosis, Chicago, 1961, Year Book Medical Publishers, Inc., pp. 3-212.

Squire, L. F.: Fundamentals of roentgenology, Cambridge, Massachusetts, 1964, Harvard University Press.

RECOMMENDED READINGS

Etter, L. E.: Roentgenography and roentgenology of the middle ear and mastoid process, Springfield, Illinois, 1965, Charles C Thomas, Publishers.

Orley, A.: Neuroradiology, Springfield, Illinois, 1949, Charles C Thomas, Publisher.

Paul, L. W., and Juhl, J. H.: The essentials of roentgen interpretation, New York, 1964, Hoeber Medical Division, Harper & Row, Publishers, pp. 241-297, 781-812.

ADDITIONAL READINGS

Davidoff, L. M., and Dyke, C. G.: The normal encephalogram, Philadelphia, 1946, Lea & Febiger.

Pendergrass, E. P., Schaeffer, J. P., and Hodes, P. J.: The head and neck in roentgen diagnosis, Springfield, Illinois, 1956, Charles C Thomas, Publisher.

Samuel, E.: Clinical radiology of the ear, nose and throat, New York, 1952, Paul B. Hoeber.

INDEX

A

Abdomen, 68-139
  basic concepts of, 68-89
  gastrointestinal system in, 109-119
  genitourinary system in, 122-138
  hepatopancreatic system in, 105-109
  lymphatic system and spleen in, 119-122
  musculoskeletal system in, 89-105
Abdominal contents, study of, 104-105
Abnormalities
  in appendicular skeleton, 164-179
  in articular components of appendicular areas, 156-164
  of gastrointestinal system, 109-119
    radiopacity of intestinal tract in, 116
  of genitourinary tract, 122-138
  of heart, 26-45
  of musculoskeletal system, 19-25, 89-105
    combined, in configurations, 143
    in components of appendicular areas, 164-179
  of respiratory system, 51-61
  of spine and spinal cord, 89-105
Abscess of respiratory structures of neck, 205
Accessory kidneys, 133
Accessory lobes of lungs, 51
Accessory spleens, 74, 122
Accessory ventricles, 243, 246
Achalasia, 61, 62
Achondroplasia, 173-175
Acromegaly, 151
  and articular components of appendicular areas, 157, 162
  chest films and, 22, 25
  and contour of bone, 175
  and paranasal sinuses, 224
Adenoma
  parathyroid, 89, 208
  thyroid, 208
  villus, 115
Aditus, 241
Adrenals, study of, 122, 124
Air-fluid level of paranasal sinuses, 222
Alignment
  of atlanto-occipital and atlantoaxial articulations, 200-201
  of cervical spine, 180, 191-192, 196
  of lumbar spine, 69
  of skeletal system
    appendicular, 176

Alignment—cont'd
  of skeletal system—cont'd
    changes in, 22, 24
  of spinal canal, 181
  of thoracic and lumbar spine in scoliosis, 90, 93
Anatomy of mastoids, 231
Anemia
  and paranasal sinuses, 224
  sickle cell, 214
Aneurysms, 151
  of vascular structures of brain, 246, 248, 251, 252
Angiocardiography, 44, 45
Angiomas, 147-148, 156
  of thymus and lymph nodes, 65
Anomalies
  of extremities, congenital, 176-177, 178
  of vertebrae, 93-95, 100
Aorta, 45-47
  atheromatous disease and, 208
  coarctation of, 17, 19, 47
  and deformity of esophagus, 62
  dilatation of, 47
  and great vessels, basic concepts of, 8
  hypoplastic, 47
Aortic insufficiency, 31, 32
Aortic valvular stenosis, 47
Appendicular areas, 140-179
  articular components in, 156-164
  basic concepts, 140-144
  skeletal components in, 164-179
  soft tissue component in, 144-156
Arm, projections of, 145
Arterial distortion in brain, 250
Arteries
  cerebral, 246-252
  in extremities, obstruction of, 156
  intracranial, 189
  in neck, 183
  opacification of, 147, 150, 151
  pulmonary, 45, 47-49
  renal, opacification of, 130
Arteriography
  of extremities, 147, 150, 151
  of genitourinary system, 130-131, 138
Arteriosclerosis and kidney function, 125
Arteriosclerotic plaque formation in neck vessels, 208, 209
Arteriovenous shunt in brain, 248, 251

253

Routine films—cont'd
  of skeletal system, 19
Rupture
  of blood vessel in brain, 250
  of viscera, 105

S

Sarcoid tumors, lymph node enlargement in, 66
Sarcoma
  Ewing's, 170
  metastatic osteogenic, and respiratory system, 54
  osteogenic, 174
Scarring of esophagus, 205
Scleroderma, 112, 113, 147-148
  esophagus and, 62
Scoliosis, 89-91, 93, 191, 193
  skeletal system and, 22
  skull films and, 213
  of spine and right atrial enlargement, 39
  types of, 69
Segmentation of lungs, 9, 49, 51
Semicircular canals, 238
Seminal vesicles
  basic concepts of, 76-77
  study of, 132-133
Shoulder, projections of, 145
Sickle cell anemia, 214
Silhouette sign, 61
Silicosis, 51
Silver fork deformity of wrist, 165
Sinuses
  paranasal
    basic concepts of, 184-185
    opacification of, 226, 227
  pyriform, 202-204
Sinusitis, 225
Size
  of aorta and great vessels, 8
  of cervical spine, 180-181
  of cervical vertebrae, 194
  of digestive system structures in neck, 182
  of endocrine structures in neck, 182
  of facial bones and orbits, 185, 226
  of heart, 7
    changes in, 26-32
  of intracranial nervous system structures, 188
  of intracranial vascular structures, 189
  of joint space, 141-142
  of kidney, 138
  of liver, 70, 105-106
    and spleen, 121
  of lung, 9
  of lymphatic system, 74
    in neck, 183
  of mastoids, 186, 238
  of orbits, 185, 226
  of pancreas, 71, 106-107
  of paranasal sinus structures, 184-185
  of petrous pyramid and middle ear, 187
  of pleura or hila, 10
  of reproductive system, 77
  of respiratory system, changes in, 51-54, 55
  of skeletal components of appendicular areas, 171, 173, 175

Size—cont'd
  of skeletal system, 143
    changes in, 22, 25
  of skull, 213, 215, 216
  of skull structures, 184
  of soft tissue, 141
    structures, 151
  of spinal canal, 194, 197, 200
  of spleen, 74
  of thymus, lymph nodes, and neurofibrous tissues, changes in, 10
  of urinary system, 75
    structures, 131
  of vascular structures
    of brain, 248, 251
    in neck, 183
Skeletal age, 164, 167
Skeletal components of appendicular areas, 164-179
Skeletal system, 19-26; *see also* Musculoskeletal system
  in appendicular areas, 164-179
    basic concepts of, 142-143
  basic concepts of, 6
Skin, margination of, 154-155
Skull, 210-216
  base of, 200
  basic concepts of, 183-184
Small bowel, proximal, projections of, 82
Small bowel series, 71, 109, 112-119
Small pulmonary vessels, 8
Small vena cavae, 8
Soft tissue
  abnormal spaces in, 151
  basic concepts of, 140-141
  calcifications of, in articular components, 156, 158-159
  components of, in appendicular areas, 144-156
  mass of, in femur, 174
Spasm
  of muscles, chest films and, 22
  of vascular structures of brain, 248
Sphenoid bone, 228-229, 230
Spina bifida, 93
Spinal canal
  cervical, study of, 194, 197, 200
  evaluation of, 181
Spinal cord, 100-103
Spinal discs, evaluation of, 69-70
Spinal segments, number of, 69
Spine
  cervical, 191-200
    evaluation of, 180
  lumbar; *see* Lumbar spine
  scoliosis of, and right atrial enlargement, 39
Spleen, 73-74, 119-122
  contrast studies of, 85-86
Splenoportography, 78, 86
Spondylolysis, 102-104
Spongiosa, 164
Spur formation of cervical vertebrae, 206, 207
Stapes, 241
Starvation and absence of fat layer, 104
Stenosis
  aortic valvular, 47